Natasha da Silva Leitão
M. Luiza M. A. Frigerio
Luciana Corrêa

Effect of propolis gel in the treatment of prosthetic stomatitis

Natasha da Silva Leitão
M. Luiza M. A. Frigerio
Luciana Corrêa

Effect of propolis gel in the treatment of prosthetic stomatitis

A clinical and cytological assessment

ScienciaScripts

Cover image: www.ingimage.com

This book is a translation from the original published under ISBN 978-3-330-76698-3.

Publisher:
Sciencia Scripts
is a trademark of
Dodo Books Indian Ocean Ltd. and OmniScriptum S.R.L publishing group

120 High Road, East Finchley, London, N2 9ED, United Kingdom
Str. Armeneasca 28/1, office 1, Chisinau MD-2012, Republic of Moldova, Europe
Managing Directors: Ieva Konstantinova, Victoria Ursu
info@omniscriptum.com

Printed at: see last page
ISBN: 978-620-8-55180-3

SUMMARY

CHAPTER 1

INTRODUCTION

Increasingly, health care, including that related to the oral health of elderly people, is undergoing changes associated with different conditions. These changes include the use of tobacco and alcohol, tooth loss, iatrogenesis caused by the use of prostheses made in disregard of biological principles, as well as systemic problems common to this population. The ageing process itself can favour the installation of lesions with consequent alterations to the oral tissues (1).

In developing countries such as Brazil, a large number of elderly people are toothless and therefore need complete dentures (PTs). According to data from the "Smiling Brazil" government project, which assessed tooth loss based on the need for prostheses in patients aged between 65 and 74, 92.7% of the population needed some kind of dental prosthesis (2).

Mucosal lesions related to the use of complete dentures (PT) can be attributed to acute or chronic reactions, associated with the presence of biofilm adhered to the base of the prosthesis, or as a result of damage caused by wear and inadequate contours of the prosthesis. Prophetic stomatitis (PS) is a chronic inflammatory process of the oral mucosa, associated with the use of dentures, and is a prevalent problem in elderly users of removable dentures (3). It affects around 58% of maxillary PT users in Brazil (1) and is most often characterised by a lack of symptoms. Its aetiology is multifactorial (4, 5) and is associated with different species of *Candida* (6), which can make it a debilitating oral disease, since the continuous ingestion or aspiration of microorganisms from the prosthesis biofilm exposes patients, especially those who are immunocompromised or elderly, to infections (7).

The treatment of PE consists of a combination of topical or systemic antifungals, guidance for the patient on hygienising the prosthesis and checking whether it needs to be replaced. The most commonly used antifungals are nystatin, amphotericin B, miconazole and fluconazole (8).

Despite the availability of a variety of antifungal drugs for the treatment of PE, the poor efficacy of the therapy is often observed, due to the high recurrence of the infection and the resistance of microorganisms to certain antimicrobial agents. Therefore, the development of new therapies for the local treatment of oral infections, as well as PE, is of great relevance (9).

In recent decades, there has been a growing use of natural products to prevent oral diseases. This is especially valuable in Brazil, where biodiversity, representing 25% of the world's flora, favours phytotherapy. Among the natural products recently studied, propolis has stood out for its pharmacological properties of medical and dental interest, which suggest its possible use in the local treatment of PE (10).

Propolis is a resinous substance collected by bees from the buds and exudates of plants and used to build and repair the hive (10). Its chemical composition includes flavonoids, aromatic acids, esters, aldehydes, ketones, terpenoids, phenylpropanoids, steroids, amino acids, polysaccharides, hydrocarbons, fatty acids and other compounds in small quantities (11, 12).

Of all these groups of compounds, the one that has certainly attracted the attention of researchers is the group of flavonoids, to which pharmacological properties are attributed (13). These properties include antibacterial (14, 15), antifungal (16, 17), antiprotozoal (18), antiviral (19), antitumour (20), immunomodulatory (21), anti-inflammatory (22) among many other therapeutic properties (23).

In view of the various pharmacological activities of propolis, its use in the local treatment of PE *is* suggested, as evidenced by the studies by Ota et al. (16) who observed a reduction in the number of *Candida albicans, Candida tropical is, Candida krusei and Candida guilliermondii* in the saliva of PT patients who used hydroalcoholic propolis extract. (24, 25) who showed the inhibition of *Candida sp.* colonisation in PT patients with PE, as well as the clinical efficacy of propolis gel in patients with PE, when compared to Daktarin® (miconazole gel).

In view of the difficulties and various factors that interfere with the treatment of PE with antifungal agents, it is necessary to use other alternatives that may be more effective in treating this infection, taking into account the side effects for the patient. In view of the above, this study set out to evaluate the effect of propolis gel in the treatment of PE in elderly users of maxillary PT and to compare the results with nystatin 100,000 IU suspension. The evaluation used clinical criteria and cytological tests at four different times.

CHAPTER 2

LITERATURE REVIEW

2.1 PROSTHETIC STOMATITIS

2.1.1 Nomenclature, Definition and Classification

In the literature, PE is understood as an inflammatory process of the oral mucosa associated with the use of removable prostheses (8). It can also be referred to as erythematous candidiasis (26), denture wound (26-28), denture stomatitis associated with *Candida sp.* (29), denture-induced stomatitis (7), oral candidiasis associated with the use of dentures (7), chronic atrophic candidiasis (28, 30), among other names.

According to Newton (31), PE can be described according to the clinical appearance, distribution and extent of inflammation of the palate mucosa, and can be classified into three types: I, II and III. Type I refers to localised hyperemic spots; type II to diffuse erythema in areas of the palatal mucosa; and type III is characterised by a hyperplastic reaction, sometimes associated with atrophic areas, and is called papillary hyperplasia.

Among the classifications derived from Newton's classification are those proposed by Budtz-Jorgensen and Bertram (32) and Bergendal and Isacsson (33). Budtz-Jorgensen and Bertram (32) adapted the terminology by calling type I PE simple localised inflammation, type II simple generalised inflammation and type III granular inflammation. Bergendal and Isacsson (33) included variations such as diffuse and papillary for atrophic and hyperplastic PE, respectively.

Barbeau et al. (6) modified Newton's classification, taking into account the extent of the inflammation. The modifications consisted of creating subclasses for types II and III PE: subclass A, when the inflammation affected one or two quadrants of the palate; or subclass B, if the inflammation was present in more than two quadrants of the palate. Thus, Newton's classification would determine the type of PE, while the subclasses would be related to the extent of the inflammatory process.

Newton's classification has been widely used in studies on PE. However, this classification tends to generate conflicts when researchers try to establish a relationship between the type of PE and the microbiological findings (8).

2.1.2 Prevalence

Studies on the prevalence of PE lead to different conclusions, depending on variations in methodology, different diagnostic methods and the sample. Arendorf and Walker (8) reported that the prevalence of PE ranges from 11% to 67%, depending on the population studied.

Shulman et al. (34) researched a representative sample of a population in the United States of America during the Third National Health and Nutrition Examination Survey (Third NHANES). The study included 33,994 individuals, 17,235 of whom underwent a dental examination, 3,450 of whom were users of some type of removable prosthesis. The prevalence of OW among these denture wearers was 28 per cent.

Studies conducted in Slovenia, Turkey and Spain reported a prevalence of PE in 14.7 per cent, 19.6 per cent and 18.5 per cent, respectively, of PT users (35-37).

A number of epidemiological studies have been carried out in Brazil. Pires et al. (38) showed that the incidence of PE in PT users in Piracicaba, São

Paulo, was 50.6%. Marchini et al. (39) observed the occurrence of PE in 42.4% of PT users treated at the University of Mogi das Cruzes, in the state of São Paulo. Freitas et al. (1) found that 57.2% of non-institutionalised elderly PT users in rural areas of western Minas Gerais had PE. In an epidemiological study in São Francisco, Sergipe, PE proved to be the most common oral lesion in users of removable prostheses (40). Another study of institutionalised elderly people in Belo Horizonte found a 15.2% incidence of PE (41).

PE has been shown to be more common in women (4, 38, 42-46). However, there are studies that show a relationship between the male gender and the presence of PE (47-49). Other studies do not establish any relationship between the disease and gender (6, 50, 51).

The studies by Baran and Nalçaci (52), Evren et al. (53), da Silva et al. (40) and Mandali et al. (54) showed a higher prevalence of PE with increasing age in PT users. Abaci et al. (49) pointed out that the relationship between advancing age and PE is due to the fact that the elderly are the biggest users of prostheses. The limitations imposed by age could be responsible for a reduction in oral hygiene care.

2.1.3 Signs and Symptoms

When present, signs and/or symptoms can appear in the form of redness and/or bleeding, swelling, a painful sensation, halitosis, an unpleasant taste and dry mouth (4, 45). However, PE is usually asymptomatic (8).

2.1.4 Diagnosis

To diagnose PE, clinical signs should be considered, such as changes in the colour and texture of the mucosa, as well as symptoms, when present. Among the tests requested are culture, cytopathological, histological or serological tests (55). According to Budtz-Jorgensen (56), culture and exfoliative cytology are the most important tools for diagnosing PE.

Conventional exfoliative cytology is a simple, quick and cheap method that consists of collecting epithelial cells by scraping the mucosa with a wooden or metal spatula or brush, which are then rubbed on a glass slide to be fixed in absolute alcohol and stained with Papanicolaou or Periodic Acid Schiff (PAS) (55).

According to the studies by Budtz-Jorgensen et al. (56) and Lemos et al. (57), cytopathology should be carried out on the oral lesion as well as the prosthesis, since the smears from patients with PE prepared from the surface of maxillary PTs showed a higher number of *Candida sp.* cells than those taken from the palatal mucosa. Swabs taken from the mucosa of the palate, dorsum of the tongue and PTs of patients affected by PE are mostly characterised by the presence of intermediate, inflammatory cells, hyphae, spores and bacteria (46, 58-60).

The therapeutic test is a widely used diagnostic measure whenever signs and symptoms compatible with PE are reported. It consists of prescribing topical antifungals and, if the lesion regresses after treatment, which varies from seven to 14 days, it can be said that the PE was associated with *Candida sp.* Other diagnostic methods available are culture, which has the disadvantage of delaying the result, and histopathological examination, which is used to diagnose chronic hyperplastic candidiasis (61).

2.1.5 Etiopathogenesis

The etiology of PE is currently believed to be multifactorial. Predisposing factors include: xerostomia, hypersensitivity to the prosthesis material (62), diabetes and other endocrine disorders, immunological alterations (28, 32, 63), prolonged use of corticosteroids (28, 64), chemotherapy and radiotherapy (28, 63, 65), use of psychotropic and hyposalivatory drugs, as well as nutritional deficiencies of vitamin B12 (28, 34), folic acid (34) and iron (66).

Prosthesis-related factors include lack of retention, which leads to trauma or irritation of the oral mucosa, age of the prosthesis, inadequate intermaxillary relationship, lack of care with oral hygiene and/or the prosthesis, pathogenic microbial infection, as well as continuous use of prostheses (28, 34, 67).

However, it should be noted that continuous use (45), sleeping with dentures (32, 48, 59, 63, 66, 68-70), poor hygiene (32, 38, 69-72) and colonisation by *Candida sp.* (4, 38, 43, 49, 66, 72, 73) are the main risk factors for developing PE.

Oliveira (74) assessed the relationship between the presence of PE and traumatic factors related to PTs, such as: occlusion, vertical occlusion dimension, retention, as well as dynamic and static stability, in addition to qualitative factors related to oral and prosthesis hygiene, continuous use, conservation, age and number of prostheses used and length of time edentulous. The study sample consisted of 116 bimaxillary PT wearers with or without PE. It was observed that functional and qualitative factors were not responsible for the frequency of PE, although they may be a facilitator for its development.

Emami et al. (66) reported that some conditions promote the overgrowth of opportunistic pathogenic yeasts such as *Candida sp.* Such conditions would be: the habit of sleeping with the prosthesis as well as its continuous use, associated with the local conditions of the mucosa, which is under the prosthesis, the low oxygen pressure, the low pH, the composition of the biofilm that coats the prosthesis, the accumulation of desquamative epithelial cells, as well as the absence of the effects of the "cleansing" carried out by saliva and tongue.

Colonisation by *Candida sp.* has been considered the main etiological factor in PE, as observed in the studies by Ramage et al. (4), Pires et al. (38), Figueiral et al. (43), Abaci et al. (49), Emami et al. (66), Coco et al. (70), Kulak et al. (72), Oliveira et al. (73), Cahn (75), Butdz-Jorgensen et al. (76), Zomorodian et al. (77), who isolated strains *of Candida sp.* in the oral mucosa, saliva and prosthesis biofilm, as well as on the internal surface of the PT of patients affected by the disease.

The adherence *of C. albicans* to the acrylic of the prosthesis is considered to be the first step in the pathogenesis of PE (4). This adhesion can occur with or without the formation of biofilm at the base of the PT (78). Although the mechanisms by which *Candida sp.* adheres to acrylic surfaces are unknown, some factors have been described. The roughness of the internal surface of the prosthesis, the surface energy of the microorganisms, the surface energy of the acrylic resin base material (79, 80), the hydrophobicity of the cell surface (79, 81) and the role of saliva (82) are some of the factors that could influence this adhesion mechanism.

PT has been considered a reservoir that enables biofilm formation (6, 38, 66, 83). The biofilm has a complex composition, involving gram-positive bacteria (30), such as *Streptococcus sanguis, Streptococcus gordonii, Streptococcus oralis, Streptococcus anginosus*, staphylococci and bacilli such as *Actinomyces*, predominantly, followed by *Lactobacillus;* and fungal blastospores, hyphae and pseudohyphae, with *C. albicans* being *the* most prevalent species. The latter colonises around 50 to 60% of PT users with PE, compared to healthy individuals (6, 38, 66, 70, 72, 76, 83).

Other *Candida* species such as *C. glabrata, C. tropicalis, Candida parapsilosis, Candida krusei, Candida pseudotropicalis, Candida dubliniensis and C. guilliermondi* have been found in patients with PE, *albeit* in lower prevalence than *C. albicans.* As a result of these findings, it is believed that these yeasts play some pathogenic role in PE (1,4, 43, 84).

C. albicans is an opportunistic pathogen, isolated in 30% to 40% of healthy adults, and in 50% to 60% of people who wear removable prostheses (49, 85). The virulence factor of *C. albicans* consists of phenotypic switching, i.e. its ability to present colony morphotypes such as mycelium and hyphae. The hyphae are more virulent and invasive due to their ability to adhere to the epithelial tissue and penetrate the host's cells. In PE lesions, invasion of the superficial oral epithelium is a striking feature, accompanied by the destruction and loss of these cells (86). In the studies by Budtz-Jorgensen et al. (76), Aguirre (46) and Lemos (57), a greater presence of *Candida* sp. hyphae was observed in swabs of the palatal mucosa and the internal surface of the PT of patients with PE. It has also been hypothesised that *C. albicans* hyphae may adhere to and penetrate the cracks in the surface of the prosthesis, thus becoming more invasive to the oral mucosa (4, 30).

Emani (66) found that the biofilm formed on the surface of PT can have an irritating effect on the palatal mucosa, favouring the installation of an inflammatory process, which in turn can modify the adhesion molecules as well as the surface structures of the host's mucosal cells. This succession of changes can favour the adhesion of pathogens. This finding would justify the results found in the studies by Al-Dwairi et al. (51), Emami et al. (87) and Dagistan et al. (88) in which the prolonged use of PT, the extent of the inflammatory process on the mucosa and a lack of hygiene would be important risk factors for the colonisation of mucosal surfaces by *Candida sp.* (49).

2.1.5 Treatment

Various treatments have been proposed for PE, but there is no consensus in the literature as to which would be the most effective. The therapeutic strategies adopted include the use of topical or systemic antifungal drugs, antiseptic agents and microwave irradiation. Another resource would be the use of lasers and the mechanical elimination of biofilm present on the internal surface of the prosthesis, as well as on the oral mucosa (63, 89, 90).

2.1.5.1 Antifungals

The use of the antifungal polyenes nystatin and amphotericin B, imidazole, miconazole and fluconazole constitutes the standard therapy for PE, according to Salerno et al. (91).

The antifungal regime for local treatment includes mouthwashes of nystatin or amphotericin B suspension. Nystatin ointment and miconazole gel should be applied to the inner surface of the PT. The entire antifungal regime should be maintained three to four times a day for two to four weeks. Suspension treatment requires the removal of dentures so that a higher concentration of the drug reaches the mucosa (92).

Nystatin is commonly used to treat PE, as it eliminates yeasts and reduces clinical signs. However, once treatment is stopped, yeast colonisation and the swollen appearance return to levels similar to those found before treatment (93).

The polyenes, nystatin and amphotericin B, bind to ergosterol, which is present in the plasma membrane, in order to cause the membrane to rupture. This binding favours the release of the intracellular content and promotes cell death. Substances with these characteristics are classified as broad-spectrum fungicides. It should be noted that both amphotericin B and nystatin have an unpleasant taste and may cause gastrointestinal side effects such as nausea, vomiting and diarrhoea. In the case of amphotericin B, there is a risk of toxicity to the renal, cardiovascular and neurological systems (67).

Dorocka-Bobkowska et al. (94) evaluated, *in vitro*, the effect of three polyene antifungals: amphotericin B, nystatin and natamycin on the adherence of *C. albicans* and *C. glabrata* to cancer cells. The authors observed that the polyenes reduced the adhesion of *Candida sp.,* however, the polyenes did not demonstrate efficacy in reducing *Candida sp.* already adhered to the cells.

Geerts et al. (95) incorporated Micostatin® into the tissue conditioner Viscogel and observed a reduction in the yeast count present in the saliva of PT users with clinical signs of PE. The authors observed that the reduction in yeasts occurred up to the fourth day in patients who received a new PT plus Viscogel. However, this period became seven days in those who received new PTs plus Viscogel/Micostatin®. After this period, the yeast count began to rise until it reached day 14. It was possible to observe, however, that the decrease in the yeast count was more evident when nystatin was incorporated into the tissue conditioner.

One problem that needs to be considered when using topical antifungal therapy is patient compliance. However, another problem concerns the rapid absorption of these agents in the oral cavity (9). The rapidity of the process means that drug concentrations are lower than necessary for therapy. In order to overcome this difficulty, the Dumex company has developed a varnish containing miconazole, which, when applied to the inner surface of the prosthesis, can maintain a relatively high concentration of the drug for a prolonged period (96).

Parvinen et al. (96) compared the efficacy of 2% miconazole gel applied four times a day for two weeks with a varnish containing 55mg of miconazole for a single application in the treatment of PE. The degree of erythema was assessed and microbiological samples were taken from the mucosa and prosthesis surface on days 3, 7, 14, 21, 28 and 35. The authors observed that treatment with the gel reduced the number of colonies more efficiently than the varnish, with the difference being statistically significant at all assessment times ($p<0.01$). It was also possible to see that *Candida sp.* recurred after the varnish treatment was discontinued. The authors therefore recommend reapplying the varnish after one month to maximise its mycological effect.

Dias et al. (97) investigated the efficacy of a varnish containing 55mg of miconazole in the mycological and clinical cure of PT-using patients with PE. There was an overall reduction of 88 per cent ($p<0.05$) in the number of yeasts after treatment. The average amount of yeast was significantly lower in the first week after starting therapy, however, in the third week there was an increase in the number of yeast, despite the improvement in palate erythema.

Systemic therapy has been reserved for oral infections that do not respond to topical agents. Fluconazole and itraconazole from the triazole group have added much to the treatment of this type of infection, since they affect the permeability of the *Candida sp.* membrane by interfering with ergosterol synthesis. However, it is important to bear in mind that hepatotoxicity and renal toxicity can occur with prolonged use of these drugs (98).

Fluconazole has been shown to be effective in reducing erythema and the concentration of yeast cells, although a high relapse rate has been reported after long-term treatment. Budtz-Jorgensen et al. (99) observed the eradication *of C. albicans* from the mucosa and also from the surface of the PT accompanied by a reduction in erythema. However, these observations became questionable when the amount of yeast in the smear was similar to that observed at the first stage of the study in the fourth week.

Kulak et al. (100) in a study with a sample of 45 PT users evaluated different conditions. The authors divided the 45 individuals into three groups: the first group received a 50mg tablet of fluconazole, twice a week; the second had 2% chlorhexidine applied to the PT surface, twice a day, associated with the use of fluconazole for a fortnight; and the third received only new PTs without using any type of medication. Of the three interventions, the combination of fluconazole and 2% chlorhexidine was the one that showed the best clinical results, with 54% of the individuals free of PE while 33% showed only an improvement in their clinical condition. Mycological examinations of the smears from all the patients did not show the presence of any hyphae, although blastospores remained. However, recurrence occurred in all three groups.

Arikan et al. (101) observed that the combination of fluconazole 50mg with 2% chlorhexidine, applied to the surface of the prosthesis twice a day for a fortnight, showed a reduction in the number of *Candida sp.* colonies *and* also in erythema in individuals with generalised PE when compared to those who received only fluconazole and new PT. The authors noted, however, that recurrence occurred after two weeks.

Cross et al. (29) compared the effect of fluconazole and itraconazole in the treatment of PE. The authors noted that both showed a reduction in erythema, as well as in the number of yeast colonies on the mucosa, although no mycological cure was observed. *C. albicans* was eradicated, but *C. glabrata* persisted after antifungal therapy.

Cross et al. (102) evaluated the effect of itraconazole capsules and liquids in the treatment of PE. They observed that the liquid form of itraconazole remained in higher concentration in saliva and blood than the capsule form. This did not represent any additional efficacy to the treatment, since both reduced mucosal erythema and eradicated *C. albicans,* although *C. glabrata* proved to be resistant.

Cross et al. (103) carried out a longitudinal study to assess the recurrence of PE in patients treated with itraconazole after three years of use.

The study included 22 patients who wore prostheses. Prosthesis-related parameters were assessed, such as hygiene habits, plaque index and the presence of erythema on the palate mucosa. Microbiological samples were also taken from the palate mucosa and tongue. The authors noted that after three years, four patients presented strains of C. *albicans* that were different from those presented initially, although the strains of *C. glabrata* remained unchanged. This result was attributed to the recurrence of the infection, since the treatment did not completely eradicate the strains; another factor to be considered was the PT, which was identified as the site of reinfection.

Koray et al. (104) compared the effect of fluconazole with hexetidine mouthwashes in the therapy of PE. The 61 patients selected were divided into three groups; the first was treated with fluconazole alone, in the form of Zolax 50 mg capsules, once a day; the second, with 0.1% hexetidine mouthrinses, twice a day; while the third received both fluconazole and hexetidine during the 14 days of the study. Patients in all groups showed a statistically significant reduction in the amount of *C. albicans* in saliva, lesions and PT after treatment, when compared to the results observed before treatment ($p<0.05$). However, there was no difference between the three groups when comparing the amount of *C. albicans* in saliva, lesions and PT after treatment.

Dorocka-Bobkowska and Konopka (105) compared the sensitivity of *Candida sp.* strains from individuals with PE to the antifungal drugs amphotericin B, 5-fluorocytosine, fluconazole and itraconazole. *C. albicans, C. glabrata, C. tropicalis* and C. *parapsilosis* proved to be sensitive to amphotericin B and 5-fluorocytosine. However, fluconazole and itraconazole were not effective against 5.6% and 7% of the *C. albicans* strains and 18.4% and 10.2% of the other *Candida sp.* strains.

In view of the above, it can be seen that antifungal therapy is effective in the treatment of PE, since there is a belief regarding the pathogenic role of *Candida sp.* in this disorder. However, it is advisable to associate prosthesis cleaning with the reduction of *Candida sp.* contamination on the PT surface.

What is known is that the effectiveness of antifungal treatment is limited, and recurrence can occur within a short period of time after the end of treatment (69, 100, 103, 104).

2.1.5.2 Herbal medicines

Phytotherapics are substances obtained from plants, which can be used as artisanal remedies in the form of teas, solutions, tablets, among others. The use of these plants to treat and cure illnesses is as old as the human race, and knowledge of their effects has spanned generations, playing an important scientific and historical role (106).

Brazil is a privileged country when it comes to the use of phytotherapy, as it has 25 per cent of the world's flora and a genetic heritage with great potential for the development of new medicines, corresponding to more than 100,000 species, less than 1 per cent of which have had their properties scientifically evaluated to determine a possible medicinal action (107).

In recent decades, there has been a growing use of natural products to prevent oral diseases. Several reports in the literature have shown that these products have antimicrobial activity against oral pathogens such as *C. albicans.* In addition, these natural products can play a very important role in the treatment of PE (108).

Vasconcelos et al. (109) evaluated the use of a gel containing pomegranate extract as an antifungal agent against candidiasis associated with PE. Sixty patients with PE were divided into two groups: group A used miconazole (Daktarin® gel) and group B used *P. granatum* (pomegranate) gel. Both groups used the medication three times a day for 15 days. Forty-eight hours after finishing the treatment, the patients were re-examined and a second set of samples was taken for fungal analysis. The clinical results showed a satisfactory response involving 27 and 21 individuals, from groups A and B, respectively. The absence of yeasts was observed in 25 individuals from group A and 23 from group B. It was concluded that *P. granatum* extract can be used as a topical antifungal agent for the treatment of PE.

Amanlou et al. (110), in a randomised study, evaluated the efficacy of miconazole gel at 2% compared to *Zataria multiflora* gel at 0.1% when applied four times a day for a fortnight in the treatment of PE. Twenty-four patients were included in the study and underwent clinical and microbiological examination of the palate mucosa and denture surface on days 0, 7, 14, 21 and 28 after the start of therapy. The results showed that *Zataria multiflora* gel reduced erythema on the palate surface more effectively than miconazole gel, but did not reduce the colony count on the denture surface as efficiently as miconazole.

Catalán et al. (111) identified the action of *Melaleuca alternifolia* (tea tree) oil incorporated into tissue conditioners on different *C. albicans* strains*, both in vitro* and *in vivo.* The *in vitro* evaluation of antifungal activity on *C. albicans* isolated from patients with class II PE involved three groups: a) *M. alternifoli;* b) tissue conditioners (Fitt, Lynal, Coe-Comfort) mixed with the oil and, c) tissue conditioners (Fitt, Lynal, Coe-Comfort) mixed with nystatin 100,000 IU. The *in vivo* activity involved 27 patients with class II PE distributed into three groups: *M. alternifoli* with Coe-Comfort; nystatin with Coe-Comfort; and Coe-Comfort, corresponding to the control group. Microbiological samples from the palate and denture surface were collected over a 12-day period. The *in vitro* results showed that the 0.2 ml dose of *M. alternifolia* oil *and* the combination of the oil with the tissue conditioners were effective in inhibiting C. *albicans;* on the other hand, when the conditioners were used alone, no effect was observed on the growth of C. *albicans.* However, the *in vivo* results showed that individuals treated with *M. alternifolia in* combination with
Coe-Comfort, obtained a significant reduction in palatal inflammation compared to those treated with Coe-Comfort alone ($p<0.001$). In addition, a significant inhibition of *C. albicans* growth was observed in individuals who used *M. alternifolia* associated with Coe-Comfort, compared to Coe-Comfort alone ($p=0.000004$). It was possible to conclude that *M. alternifolia* oil associated with Coe-Comfort tissue conditioner is effective in the treatment of

PE.

Paiva et al. (112) evaluated the action of the gel from the cat's claw plant, *Uncaria tomentosa*, on patients with oral candidiasis. For this assessment, 20 patients were divided into two groups: the test group, which was instructed to use *Uncaria tomentosa* gel on the lesions in the oral cavity three times a day for a period of 14 days, and the control group, which used Miconazole (Daktarin® gel) in the same way as prescribed for the test group. After the treatment period, the patients returned for a new clinical and laboratory assessment. Three of the ten patients (30 per cent) had no symptoms related to candidiasis after 14 days of treatment with *Uncaria tomentosa* gel, while the group that used Miconazole showed the disappearance of symptoms in 40 per cent of the patients. An effective action of *Uncaria tomentosa* gel was observed on the species C. *albicans, C. tropicalis* and C. *guilliermondii.* Thus, *Uncaria tomentosa* proved to be a promising phytopharmaceutical in dentistry, showing an advantage over miconazole, as it did not cause any adverse reactions in the patients, while 40 per cent of the patients in the control group (miconazole) showed undesirable reactions, such as nausea and epigastric pain.

However, further studies are needed to clarify the antifungal mechanism of the extracts under different conditions.

2.1.5.2.1 Propolis

The word propolis is derived from the Greek *pro-,* in defence, and *polis-,* city or community, i.e. in defence of the community (113). In general, propolis contains 50-60% resins and balsams, 30-40% waxes, 5-10% essential oils, 5% pollen grains, as well as microelements such as aluminium, calcium, strontium, iron, copper, manganese and small amounts of vitamins B1, B2, B6, C and E (114).

The colour of propolis depends on where it comes from. It has a range of colours from dark brown, to a greenish hue, to a reddish brown. Propolis has a characteristic odour, which can vary from one sample to another (115).

Crude propolis contains impurities such as wood, wax, pollen and dead bees, so macroscopic observation of the sample is necessary to eliminate impurities and purify the propolis before preparing the extracts. The solvents used to extract propolis are generally alcohols: methanol and ethanol. However, the most commonly used solvent is ethanol. 70% ethanol is ideal for extracting most of the active components of propolis. Water has also been used in some studies, however, it is important to note that, in general, water dissolves a small part of the propolis constituents, around 10 per cent of its weight, while 70 per cent ethanol can dissolve 50 to 70 per cent, depending on the amount of wax. Propolis extracts are prepared by maceration or, in some cases, with procedures using methanol or 96% ethanol. These extraction processes, using different solvents (methanol, ethanol or water), can extract different compounds from propolis, which can influence its pharmacological activities (Figure 2.1) (116).

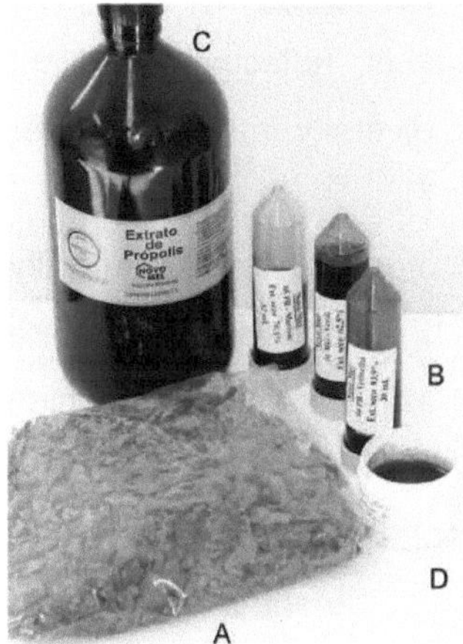

Figure 2.1 Propolis (A) raw propolis, (B) aqueous propolis extract, (C) ethanolic propolis extract, (D) propolis gel

The chemical composition of propolis is quite complex and varied, and is related to the ecology of the flora of each region visited by the bees, as well as the period during which the resin is collected. It should be emphasised that the genetic variability of queen bees also influences the chemical composition of propolis (114).

The chemical compounds in propolis include flavonoids (such as galangin, quercetin, pinocembrin and kaempferol), aromatic acids and esters, aldehydes and ketones, terpenoids and phenylpropanoids (such as caffeic and chlorogenic acids), steroids, amino acids, polysaccharides, hydrocarbons, fatty acids and various other compounds in small quantities (11). It also contains inorganic elements such as copper, manganese, iron, calcium, aluminium, vanadium and silicon (115).

Of all these groups of compounds, the one that has certainly attracted the most attention from researchers is flavonoids (117). They, as well as phenolic acids, are attributed antibacterial properties (14, 15, 118), antiviral, antioxidant (13), antifungal (16, 17), antiprotozoal (18), antitumour, immunomodulation (21), anti-inflammatory (22) and other therapeutic properties (23).

The range of pharmacological activities of propolis is greater in tropical regions of the planet and lower in temperate regions, reflecting the plant diversity of these regions; in tropical regions plant diversity is much greater than the diversity observed in temperate regions (117).

In 2000, twelve different types of Brazilian propolis were chemically characterised and classified from type 1 to 12. However, there are controversies regarding the flavonoid content of Brazilian samples, in which phenolic acids are generally much more abundant (11). Mantovani et al. (119) evaluated the chemical composition of propolis samples collected in the south and southeast regions of Brazil, and the sample from the south showed the highest amount of flavonoids in its composition, while the sample from the southeast showed the highest amount of total phenolic compounds.

Propolis is one of the few "natural remedies" that has been used for a long time by different civilisations. Although there are already reports attributing propolis to the most varied applications in folk medicine and veterinary medicine, scientific studies have corroborated the great therapeutic potential of propolis, especially with regard to anti-inflammatory, antimicrobial, antineoplastic and antioxidant activities. In addition to research and the development of new drugs, a better understanding of its properties aims to add economic value to raw propolis in order to generate an economic source for farming and self-sustainable extraction (120).

Certainly, propolis' ability to inhibit the growth of microorganisms is its best known and most scientifically proven pharmacological activity. Despite their different compositions, propolis samples from Europe are very similar to those from Brazil in terms of antimicrobial activity (121).

The antimicrobial activity of propolis is mainly attributed to flavonones, pinocembrin, the flavonol galagin and the phenylethyl ester of caffeic acid, which probably inhibit bacterial RNA-polymerase. Other components such as flavonoids, caffeic acid, benzoic acid and cinnamic acid act on the bacteria's membrane or cell wall, causing functional and structural damage (118).

The first systematic investigation into the antibacterial properties of propolis was carried out by Kikalvin in 1948 (122). This property is mainly due to the flavonoids, pinocembrin and galangin. Park et al. (123) demonstrated antibacterial activity in cultures of *Staphylococcus aureus, Bacillus subtilis, Salmonella typhimurium and Salmonella enteritides.* Antibiosis tests with propolis against ten gram-positive and 20 gram-negative bacteria found that the antibacterial activity of propolis is more effective against gram-positive bacteria (124).

Propolis has also demonstrated excellent fungistatic and fungicidal activities *in in vitro* tests with yeasts (125). Ota et al. (126) verified the influence of propolis extract on the number of *Candida sp.* present in saliva. The antifungal activity of propolis was studied in sensitivity tests on 80 strains *of Candida* species*:* 20 strains of *C. albicans,* 20 strains of *C. tropicalis,* 20 strains of *C. krusei* and 15 strains *of C. guilliermondii.* It was observed that propolis showed antifungal activity against *C. albicans, C. tropicalis, C. krusei and C. guilliermondii*, respectively. In the *in vivo* test, patients using PT who used the hydroalcoholic propolis extract showed a decrease in the number of *Candida sp- and C.* guilliermondii.

D'Aurea et al. (127) evaluated the effect of propolis extract on the virulence factors of *C. albicans.* They assessed hyphae formation, phospholipase activity and adhesion of the fungi to epithelial cells. The two propolis samples used significantly inhibited the *C. albicans* strains. In addition, the length of hyphae was reduced even with a low concentration of propolis. There was inhibition of phospholipase activity, depending on the dose and time of action; no effect was observed with regard to adhesion to oral epithelial cells and surface hydrophobicity.

Dias et al. (128) evaluated, *in vitro*, the antifungal activity of fourteen commercial samples of ethanolic and aqueous extracts of Brazilian propolis against strains of *C. albicans, C. tropicalis, C. glabrata, C. parapsilosis, C. krusei and C. guilliermondii.* Nystatin (100,000 IU), sterile distilled water and ethanol were used as positive, negative and solvent controls, respectively. The results showed that all the ethanolic extracts of propolis tested inhibited the *in vitro* growth of *Candida sp.* The aqueous extract of propolis showed little or no efficacy in inhibiting the *in vitro* growth of yeasts. In addition, the aqueous propolis extract promoted significantly smaller zones of inhibition than nystatin. Thus, the authors suggested that ethanolic extracts of propolis could be used as an alternative medicine for the treatment of fungal infections of the oral cavity, such as oral candidiasis or PE, since ethanolic extracts of propolis were more effective against *Candida sp.*

Molina (129) et al. evaluated *in vitro* the antifungal activity of natural extracts (propolis, castor bean, sage and calendula) on 20 strains of *C. albicans* isolated from the oral cavity. The results showed that the glycolic extract of propolis had fungicidal capacity for all strains *of C. albicans*, with a minimum fungicidal concentration of 3.12% for 90% of the strains. The glycolic extract of sage showed fungicidal capacity for 80 per cent of the strains, with a minimum fungicidal concentration ranging from five to 50 per cent. Calendula glycolic extract showed fungicidal activity for only 10% of the strains. Castor bean extract showed no fungicidal activity for any strain. It was concluded that propolis extract was the most effective, showing antifungal activity for all the *C. albicans* strains evaluated.

Given the activities of propolis, some studies such as those by Ceschel et al. (9), Santos et al. (24), Santos et al. (25), Gomes et al. (130), and Casaroto et al. (108) have suggested its use in the treatment of oral infectious diseases, since the use of topical agents has the disadvantage of an initial burst effect followed by a rapid decrease in concentration due to salivary flow and tissue mobility.

Thus, buccal mucoadhesive formulations, which control the release of the drug, are expected to overcome the problems as observed in the study by Ceschel et al. (9). This study developed a mucoadhesive topical formulation containing ethanolic extract of propolis and then carried out an *in vivo* test on ten volunteers for eight hours in order to assess the mucoadhesive behaviour and comfort of the formulation. The authors noted that the gel had technological characteristics such as: high solubility of propolis, absence of ethanol which has irritating actions on the oral mucosa and the ability to absorb the flow of propolis through the mucosa. The *in vivo* evaluation of the mucoadhesive gel revealed adequate comfort without causing irritation during the study period, and it was also accepted by the volunteers.

Gomes et al. (130), in an *in vitro* study, evaluated the antimicrobial activity of a propolis adhesive formulation, using the agar diffusion method with different concentrations of propolis (5%, 10%, 15% and 20%), against seven oral pathogens: C. *albicans, C. tropicalis, Streptococcus mutans, Staphylococcus aureus, Enterococcus faecalis, Actinomyces israelli, Actinobacillus actinomycetemcomitans.* It was observed that the 20% propolis ointment had statistically different growth inhibition zones to the 5% propolis ointment for all the microorganisms tested ($p<0.05$). For all the concentrations of propolis tested in the study, the *Candida* strains were more susceptible to propolis than to 5% nystatin (positive control), and all the bacteria tested were more susceptible to 20% propolis ointment compared to the positive control

(1% tetracycline) ($p<0.05$). Thus, the authors concluded that the antimicrobial action observed in this new formulation makes it possible to suggest its use as an alternative therapy for infectious conditions of the oral cavity, without causing major local or systemic adverse effects.

2.1.5.2.1.1 Propolis in the treatment of prosthetic stomatitis

As observed in the aforementioned studies, Gomes et al. (130) and Dias et al. (128) suggest propolis as an alternative treatment for PE, since existing therapies do not prevent recurrence of the infection because they do not eradicate *Candida sp.* strains.

Santos et al. (24) analysed the topical therapeutic effect of green Brazilian propolis extract on oral candidiasis in patients using PT compared to the control group, which used nystatin. The results indicated that there was a similar regression between the patients who were treated with propolis extract and nystatin. The researchers believe that the therapeutic method used in this research is effective in treating oral candidiasis associated with PE.

Silva et al. (131) analysed the influence of nystatin, fluconazole and propolis orobase gel on the surface of acrylic resins over a 14-day period. The results showed that roughness increased for both acrylic resins, although they did not differ from each other ($p>0.05$). The authors concluded that antifungal agents can interfere with the surface properties of acrylic resin when it is associated with *Candida sp.* adhesion.

Santos et al. (25), in a pilot study, clinically evaluated the efficacy of a new formulation of Brazilian propolis gel in patients diagnosed with PE. The study sample consisted of 30 PT-using patients who were divided into two groups: those who received treatment with Daktarin® gel and those who received Brazilian propolis gel. All patients were instructed to apply the product four times a day for one week. Patients who were treated with Daktarin® gel and Brazilian propolis gel had clinical remission of palate oedema and erythema. According to the authors, Brazilian propolis gel could be an alternative for the topical treatment of PE.

Several treatments have been proposed for PE in the literature, but its recurrence rate is high due to the lack of effective therapies for eradicating the fungus from the mucosa and, especially, the prosthesis. In view of this, the use of natural products as an alternative for the treatment and/or prevention of oral diseases can provide this effectiveness, since they have essential therapeutic characteristics for curing this infection. Propolis fits into this context, as it has anti-inflammatory, antibacterial and antifungal activities. In order to help elucidate this issue, this study aims to use a mucoadhesive propolis gel for the treatment of PE, as well as evaluating its clinical and cytological effect.

CHAPTER 3

PROPOSAL

3.1 GENERAL OBJECTIVE

To evaluate the efficacy of propolis gel compared to nystatin suspension in the treatment of PE, by means of clinical and cytological analysis.

3.2 SPECIFIC OBJECTIVES

- Characterise the cytological findings of the palatine mucosa and the internal surface of the PT before the intervention;
- Evaluate and compare the clinical effect of the treatments on the palate mucosa before and after the intervention; e,
- To assess the presence or absence of epithelial cells, inflammatory cells, fungi and/or bacteria on the palate mucosa and the inner surface of the PT, and to compare the findings before and after the interventions.

CHAPTER 4

CASUISTRY - MATERIAL AND METHODS

This study sought to clinically and through exfoliative cytology evaluate PE in elderly PT users and the effect of propolis gel as an alternative therapy for this infection.

The selected patients were divided into two groups. One group applied propolis gel to the inner surface of the maxillary PT, while the other group mouthwashed with nystatin four times a day for a period of fourteen days.

These patients were diagnosed as to the type of PE and underwent exfoliative cytology examinations at four different times. Questionnaires were administered to assess cognitive function and provide demographic data including common complaints, smoking, time and habit of prosthesis use and hygiene.

4.1 CASUISTICS

A total of 160 individuals were assessed, including 32 edentulous patients with maxillary PT with PE who voluntarily attended the Envelhecer Sorrindo Programme Clinic of the Prosthetics Department at the University of São Paulo School of Dentistry (FOUSP) between September 2011 and June 2012.

This research was approved by the FOUSP Research Ethics Committee under protocol 191/10. The Informed Consent Form was duly given to all patients, informing them of the purpose of the research, the methods of work and treatment. Participation took place spontaneously after being informed of all the details of the study.

the content of the study, the risks and benefits, with all relevant questions answered. Patients had the option of agreeing to take part in the study or not, and were completely free to withdraw from the study at any time they saw fit. The confidentiality of the information obtained was preserved throughout the process.

The ethical purposes related to this work are based on Resolution 196/96 of the Brazilian legislation issued by the Ministry of Health (132), which directs all research involving human beings to respect the principles of autonomy, beneficence, non-maleficence and justice, in an attempt to preserve the citizenship and dignity of the research participants.

4.2 MATERIAL

The materials used to carry out the research were:

- Anamnesis form;
- Mini Mental State Examination (MMSE);
- *Cytobrush,* (Kolplast Comercial Industrial do Brasil Ltda, São Paulo, SP, Brazil);
- Propolis gel (Bioactive Tecnologia em Polímeros LTDA) (Figure 4.1);
- Suspension of nystatin 100,000 IU (Generic from Laboratório Teuto Brasileiro) (Figure 4.2);
- 95% alcohol;
- Blade holder;
- Pap smear;
- PAS staining;
- Glass slides for microscopy 26x76mm matt polished (Precision);
- 24X60 coverslips (Precision); e,
- Binocular microscope model Olympus CH2 (Olympus®, Japan).

4.2.1 Propolis gel composition

The gel (Figure 4.1) was supplied by the company Bioactive Tecnologia em Polímeros LTDA (São Paulo, SP, Brazil), containing 81.2 per cent copolymer of e- caprolactone, l-lactide and polyethylene glycol (Sigma-Aldrich, United States) associated with 5 per cent aqueous extract of purified brown propolis (Novomel Company, São Paulo, SP, Brazil), and supplemented with saccharin, menthol and ultrapure water (Synth, São Paulo, SP, Brazil). The gel is patented by Bioactive.

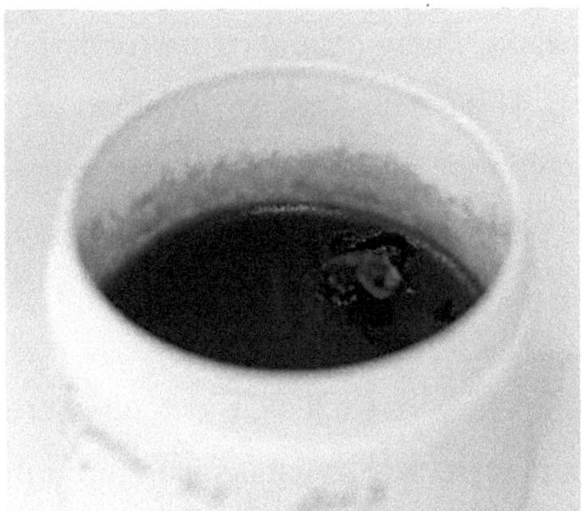

Figure 4.1 - Propolis gel

4.2.2 Composition of nystatin 100,000 IU suspension

The nystatin oral suspension (Figure 4.2), used in this study, is a generic medicine, under Law 9.787 of 1999, from the Teuto Brasileiro Laboratory. Each ml of the suspension contains nystatin (100,000 UI/ml) and glycerol, sorbitol 70%, sucrose, carboxymethylcellulose, dibasic sodium phosphate, methylparaben, propylparaben, disodium edetate, alcohol, cherry/mint flavouring and purified water as a carrier (1 ml).

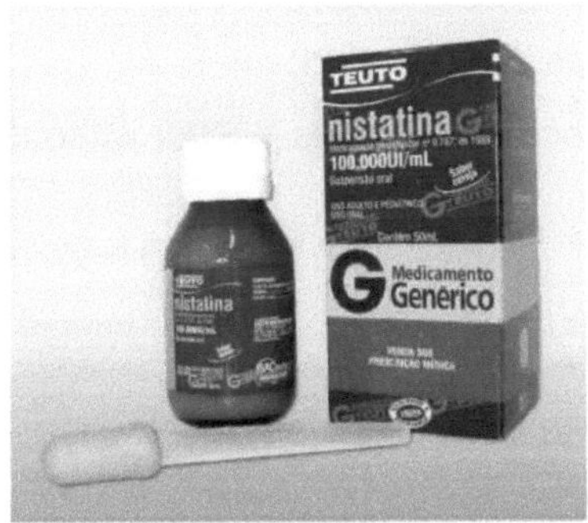

Figure 4.2 - Nystatin 100,000 IU oral suspension

4.3 METHOD

4.3.1 Study design

The study consisted of a single-blind randomised controlled clinical trial. Randomisation took place by random allocation, where patients were randomly assigned to which group they would belong. Thus, there was an envelope with green cards, which corresponded to the propolis gel group, and red cards, referring to the nystatin group. In this way, the patients were allocated to each group until the groups were complete (133).

4.3.2 Sample selection

Patients who met the study's inclusion and exclusion criteria were selected to take part in the study. All patients were clinically assessed through anamnesis and clinical examination.

4.3.2.1 Inclusion criteria

- Patients of both genders;
- Age > 60 years;
- Maxillary PT users;
- Not being under prophetic treatment;
- Have PE classes 1 and 2, according to Newton's classification, and;
- MEEM score > 25

4.3.2.2 Exclusion criteria

- Have a maxillary removable partial prosthesis (RPP), implant-supported or implant-retained;
- Present EP class 3, according to Newton's classification;
- Systemic infectious disease of any kind, acute or chronic, with or without oral manifestations;
- Malignant neoplasms of an oral nature;
- Have undergone any type of radiotherapy treatment;
- Have undergone prolonged treatment with broad-spectrum antibiotic or antifungal therapy;
- Being allergic to propolis and honey; e,
- Not consenting to take part in the study.

4.3.2.3 Nystatin group

Fifteen patients received conventional treatment with a suspension of nystatin 100,000 IU, as indicated by the manufacturer (generic Teuto Brasileiro Laboratory), which consisted of daily oral use of 5 ml every six hours for 14 days, swishing the solution around and keeping it in the mouth for one minute.

4.3.2.4 Propolis gel group

Fifteen patients had propolis gel applied to the inner surface of the maxillary PT four times a day for a period of fourteen days. Before the application, the patients were instructed to clean the PT and mucosa in the usual way. The method of application was demonstrated to each patient individually. The gel was applied with the index finger to the entire dry inner surface of the PT (24, 25).

4.4 FIELD OF STUDY

The research was carried out at the Envelhecer Sorrindo Programme outpatient clinic in the Prosthetics Department and the cytopathological analyses were carried out in the Pathology laboratory, both located at the University of São Paulo School of Dentistry (FOUSP), at Avenida Professor Lineu Prestes, 2227, Cidade Universitária, Butantã, São Paulo-SP. The propolis gel was produced and supplied by Bioactive Tecnologia em Polímeros LTDA, at Avenida Professor Lineu Prestes, 2242, Instituto de Pesquisas Energéticas e Nucleares (IPEN), Centro de Inovação, Empreendedorismo e Tecnologia (CIETEC), sala 01, Cidade Universitária - Butantã, São Paulo.

4.5 DATA COLLECTION PROCEDURES

4.5.1 Questionnaires

Data collection took place on Wednesdays at the Envelhecer Sorrindo Programme Outpatient Clinic of the Prosthetics Department at FOUSP. All participants were subjected to a questionnaire produced by the researcher in charge, which aimed to assess demographic data as well as systemic conditions, use of medication, smoking, age of the prosthesis, use and hygiene habits in relation to the PT. In addition to this questionnaire, another questionnaire called the MMSE was used to assess cognition, in order to assess whether the patients were able to assimilate the guidelines related to the study methodology.

a. Mini Mental State Examination

Patients answered questions grouped into seven categories, each designed to assess specific cognitive functions such as temporal orientation (5 points), spatial orientation (5 points), three-word recording (3 points), attention and calculation (5 points), three-word recall (3 points), language (8 points) and visual constructive capacity (1 point). The MMSE score can vary from a minimum of 0 points, which indicates the greatest degree of cognitive impairment in individuals, to a maximum total of 30 points, which corresponds to the best cognitive ability. Any score equal to or greater than 25 points (out of 30) is considered normal. These values are analysed according to the participants' level of education, with those with a score of less than 24 being considered cognitively impaired in the case of highly educated patients; those with a score of less than 18 in the case of patients with up to a medium level of education; for illiterate , scores of less than 14 already determine some degree of impairment (134).

4.3.3 Diagnosis of prosthetic stomatitis

PE was diagnosed clinically, taking into account changes in the colour and texture of the mucosa, as well as symptoms. The lesions were classified according to the criteria established by Newton (31): type I: localised inflammation or punctiform hyperemia; type II: diffuse erythema; type III: papillary hyperplasia on the palate, as seen in figure 4.3.

In order to assess the clinical response of the subjects' mucosa to the proposed treatments, during the different assessment moments, the degree of erythema was classified according to the index proposed by Budtz-Jorgensen et al. (99), which comprises four degrees: 0: no inflammation; 1: mild inflammation, 2: moderate inflammation and 3: severe inflammation.

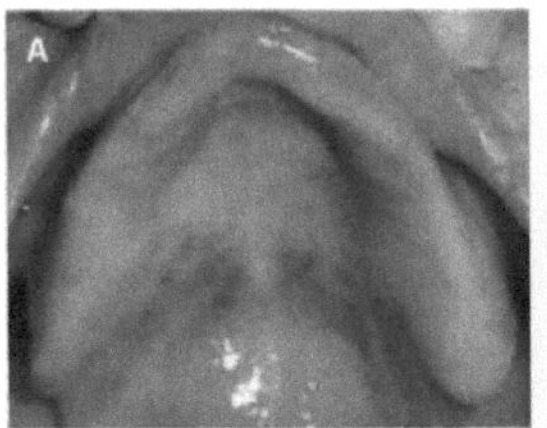 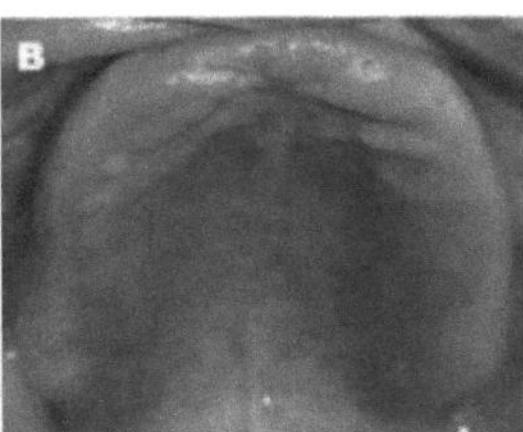 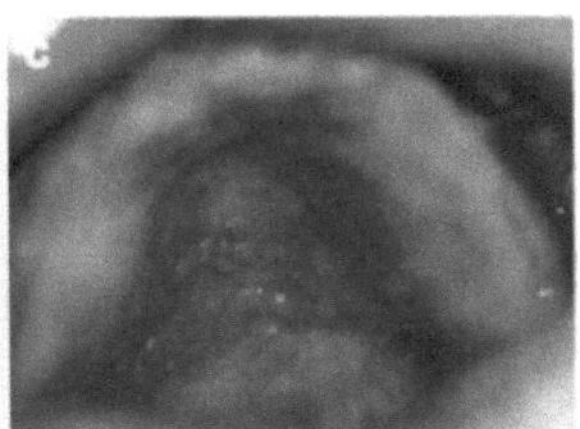

Figure 4.3 - Newton's classification (A) Type I: localised inflammation or punctiform hyperemia, (B) Type II: diffuse erythema and (C) Type III: papillary hyperplasia

4.5.3 Exfoliative cytology and laboratory processing

A *citobrush* (Kolplast Comercial Industrial do Brasil Ltda, São Paulo, SP, Brazil) was used to collect epithelial, inflammatory and microbial cells from the palatal mucosa under the PT, as well as the biofilm present on the internal surface of the maxillary PT.

Before collecting the cells, the patient mouthwashed with water to remove any necrotic or food debris that might be present on the mucosa. The toothbrush was placed in the patient's mouth until the bristles touched the erythematous area on the palatal mucosa (Figure 4.4).

The internal surface of the prosthesis was collected immediately after removing it from the patient's mouth. The brush was scrubbed,
vigorously over the surface of the PT in order to collect as much biofilm as possible (Figure 4.5).

The smear was then applied to clean, dry glass slides, which were immediately dipped in 95% alcohol and left in this solution for at least an hour (Figure 4.6).

Four slides were obtained for each patient, three from the palatal mucosa and one from the maxillary PT. The slides were labelled and accompanied by a brief clinical summary.

Collections were made before the interventions began (day 0), and 5, 7 and 14 days after the applications.

The samples were sent and processed in the laboratory for staining using the Papanicolaou and PAS techniques. All processing was carried out at FOUSP's Pathology Laboratory.

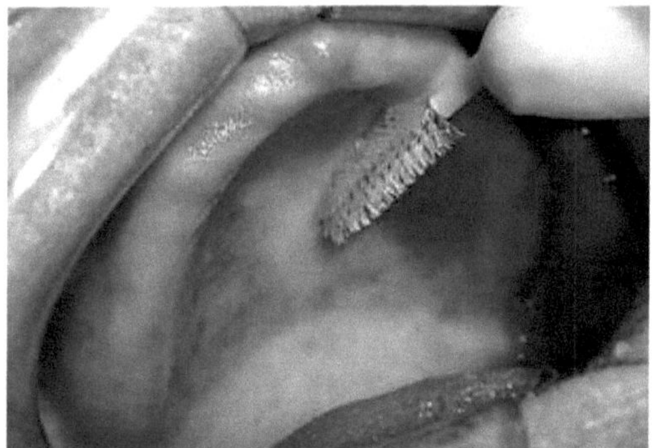

Figure 4.4 - Collecting cells from the palate mucosa with a *cytobrush*

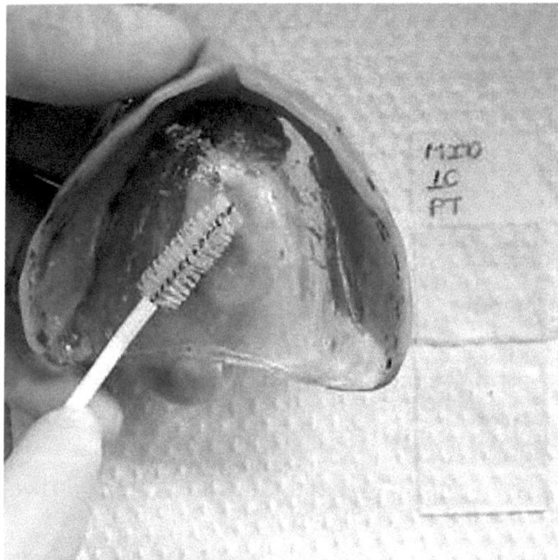

Figure 4.5 - Collection of biofilm from the inner surface of the maxillary PT with a *cytobrush*

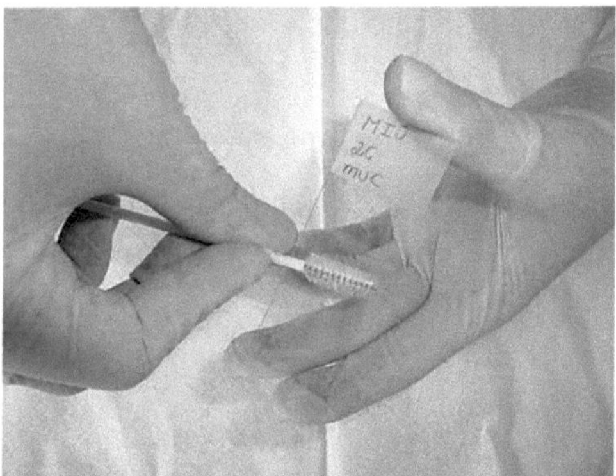

Figure 4.6 - Smear on glass slide

4.5.3.1 Papanicolaou staining

Papanicolaou staining was carried out using the Tissue-Tek DRS 2000 A-D1 machine (Sakura®), according to the FOUSP Pathology Laboratory protocol described in Table 4.1 (Figure 4.7).

Steps	Chemical substance	Procedures
1	Running water	10 dives
2	Distilled water	10-15 dives
3	Harris haematoxylin	3 minutes
4	Running water	5 minutes
5	Distilled water	2 dives
6	Absolute Alcohol	2 minutes
7	Orange G-36	15 minutes
8	Absolute Alcohol	10-15 dives
9	EA-36	15 minutes
10	Absolute Alcohol	10 dives
11	Absolute Alcohol	10 dives
12	Absolute Alcohol	10 dives
13	Absolute Alcohol	10 dives
14	50/50 Xylol and Alcohol	10-15 dives
15	Xylol I	5 minutes
16	Xylol II	5 minutes

Table 4.1 - Descriptive table of the sequence of the Papanicolaou staining technique

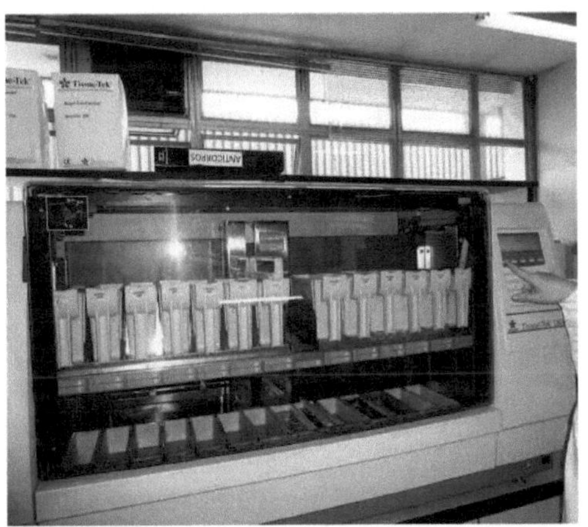

Figure 4.7 - Papanicolaou staining performed on the Tissue-Tek DRS 2000 A- D1 machine (Sakura®)

4.5.3.2 Periodic acid Schiff staining

PAS staining was carried out according to the protocol used at FOUSP's Pathology Laboratory, illustrated in Table 4.2 (Figure 4.8).

Steps	Chemical substances	Procedures
1	0.5% periodic acid	20 minutes
2	Running water	5 minutes

3	Schiff's solution	30 minutes
4	Running water	5 minutes
5	Harris haematoxylin	5 minutes
6	Running water	5 minutes
7	Alcohol 80%	5 minutes
8	90% alcohol	5 minutes
9	Absolute alcohol	3 minutes
10	Absolute alcohol	3 minutes
11	50/50 Xylol and absolute alcohol	5 dives
12	Xylol I	3 minutes
13	Xylol II	3 minutes

Table 4.2 - Descriptive table of the sequence of the PAS staining technique

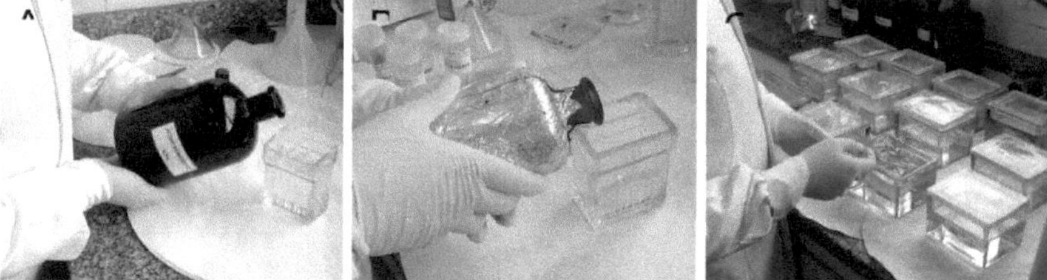

Figure 4.8 - PAS staining sequence: (A) Periodic Acid 0.5%, (B) Shiff's solution and (C) Dehydration in alcohol

4.5.3.3 Analysing the slides

After staining, the slides were analysed by light microscopy using a binocular microscope, model Olympus CH2 (Olympus®, Japan). The analyses were carried out by a single trained pathologist, who did not know the type of treatment the patient had received.

The slides were assessed for the presence of cellular alterations using a semi-quantitative analysis (abundant, moderate, scarce and absent). The data was recorded on the cytology registration form used by the FOUSP Pathology Laboratory.

4.5.3.4 Definition of cytological parameters

For the qualitative analysis, the scanning technique was used along the entire length of the slide, where the presence of mucus, inflammatory cells, red blood cells, debris, artefacts and the morphological characteristics of the epithelial cells were observed. The cytological diagnosis of PE was confirmed when the smear showed the presence of hyphae and/or pseudohyphae stained pink.

To classify the number of epithelial cells, inflammatory cells, fungi and bacteria present on each slide, the following criteria were proposed: absent, scarce, moderate and abundant.

4.6 STUDY PROTOCOL

After being included in the study, the patients underwent an anamnesis in which they were asked about their systemic condition, as well as the use of medication, the length of time they had been using PT, night-time use of the prosthesis, the form and frequency of prosthesis hygiene, as well as an assessment of the clinical picture and symptoms of PE.

The patients were then randomly divided into two groups to undergo four tests and analyses. At the first stage (day 0), the patients were diagnosed according to the type of PE by a single trained examiner, who determined whether or not the patient could be included in the sample. Subsequently, a cytopathological examination of the lesion was carried out to assess the cellular changes in the damaged mucosa. Through

Two groups were formed by simple randomisation. One group received nystatin suspension 100,000 IU and the other received propolis gel. All the patients received information about the composition, risks and benefits of the interventions, as well as instructions regarding the applications and maintenance of oral hygiene.

The patients returned 5, 7 and 14 days after the first collection, when they were again subjected to the analyses and tests described above. The tests at this stage were carried out by a second trained examiner to avoid biased results, since the first examiner knew the type of treatment the patient had received.

Patients treated with nystatin received treatment as recommended by the laboratory. Patients treated with propolis who did not show regression of the clinical picture and/or absence of hyphae in the exfoliative cytology after the end of the research protocol were also treated with nystatin.

The slides were sent to the FOUSP Pathology Laboratory to be analysed by exfoliative cytology.

4.7 DATA ANALYSES

The software used for descriptive statistics and non-parametric tests was *Statistical Package for Social Science* (SPSS), version 20.0. Quantitative measures were described using mean, standard deviation and percentage statistics, minimum (min) and maximum (max) values. The Friedman non-parametric test was used for the dependent variables in order to compare the variables between the study moments. Multiple ranking comparisons were carried out to analyse the differences between the time points. For independent samples, the Mann-Whitney non-parametric test was used to compare the findings before and after treatment, and the Chi-square test was used to compare the frequency of cytological findings on the palatal mucosa and the inner surface of the PT. The significance level of the tests was 5%, i.e. significant differences were considered when the descriptive level of the test (p-value) was less than 0.05.

CHAPTER 5

RESULTS

5.1 DEMOGRAPHIC AND CLINICAL CHARACTERISTICS OF THE SAMPLE

Figure 5.1 shows the patient recruitment diagram. Of the 160 patients eligible for the study, 37 (23.1%) had PE, but five patients did not fulfil the inclusion criteria. In the end, 30 (18.8%) patients completed the study.

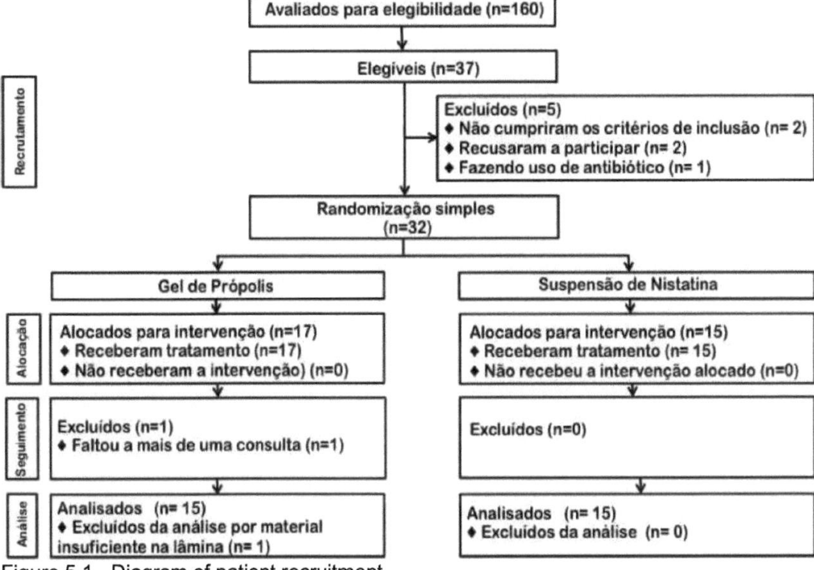

Figure 5.1 - Diagram of patient recruitment

Table 5.1 describes the demographic and clinical characteristics of the patients. The sample was made up predominantly of women with a mean age of 74.5±6.7 years. Twelve (70.0%) patients had completed primary school. Twenty-eight (93.3%) patients did not smoke and 22 (73.3%) were not social drinkers. Among the associated comorbidities, hypertension was the most prevalent (56.6%) followed by osteoporosis (26.7%).

Table 5.1 - Demographic and clinical characteristics of the sample

Variables		n=30	%
Gender	Male	4	13,3

	Female	26	86,7
Age	75±6,7; 60-87*		
Education	Illiterate	3	10,0
	Fundamental	12	70,0
	High School	3	10,0
Smoke	Smoke	2	6,6
	Doesn't smoke	28	93,3
Use of alcohol	Drinking alcohol	8	26,7
	Doesn't drink alcohol	22	73,3
Comorbidities	Hypertension	17	56,6
	Diabetes *mellitus*	3	10,0
	Depression	4	13,3
	Nephritis	4	13,3
	Renal insufficiency	1	3,3
	Kidney stones	4	13,3
	Cirrhosis	1	3,3
	Anaemia	2	6,7
	Arthritis	3	10,0
	Arthrosis	5	16,7
	Rheumatism	3	10,0
	Osteoporosis	8	26,7

*Mean ± standard deviation; minimum - maximum

The sample's risk factors for developing PE in relation to the use of PT can be seen in table 5.2.

Table 5.2 - Risk factors for PE related to the use of maxillary PT

Variables		**n=3 0**	%
Age of maxillary PT	10+15,4 (1 -50)*		
Removing the prosthesis during the day	Remove the prosthesis	5	16,7%
	Does not remove the prosthesis	25	83,3%
Sleeping with your prosthesis	Sleeps with a prosthesis	5	16,7%
	Doesn't sleep with a prosthesis	25	83,3%
Denture hygiene method	Toothbrush and water	1	3,3%
	Toothbrush and paste	26	86,7%
	Toothbrush and soap	3	10,0%
Hygiene by immersion in chemical solution	Sodium hypochlorite	6	20,0%
	Other solutions	3	10,0%
	No solution	21	70,0%
Hygiene frequency	Once	4	13,3%
	Twice	10	33,3%
	Three times	10	33,3%
	More often	6	20,0%
Use of fixative	Use fixative	3	10%
	No fixative	27	90%

*average + standard deviation (minimum-maximum value)

The mean age of the maxillary PTs was 10±15.4 years. All the patients reported removing their dentures to clean them. Twenty-five (83.3%) patients did not take their dentures out during the day and had the habit of sleeping with them in.

As for denture hygiene habits, 86.7% of patients cleaned their dentures with a toothbrush and toothpaste, while 70.0% did not immerse their dentures in a chemical solution. With regard to the frequency of denture hygiene, 33.3% sanitised twice a day and 33.3% three times.

Figure 5.2 shows the frequency of symptoms reported before the treatments proposed in the study. Nineteen (63.3%) of the 30 patients reported oral symptoms such as dry mouth, unpleasant taste, pain and loss of taste, with dry mouth (47.0%) being the most frequent symptom.

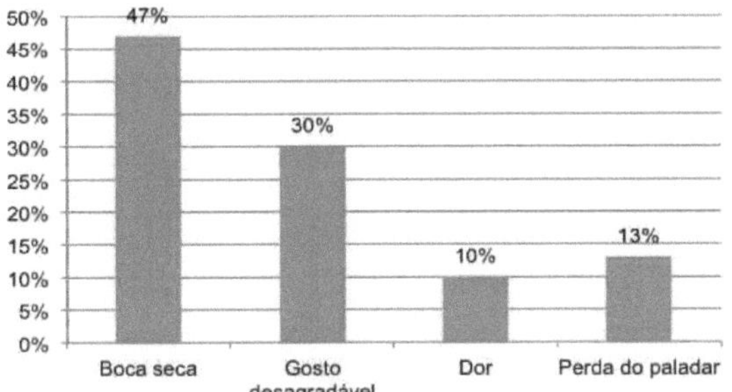

Figure 5.2 - Frequency of symptoms reported during anamnesis

5.2 EVALUATION AND CLINICAL CLASSIFICATION OF PROSTHETIC STOMATITIS

The intraoral examination revealed that 66.7% of the sample had type II PE and 36.6% had grade II erythema on day 0, as shown in figures 5.3 and 5.4.

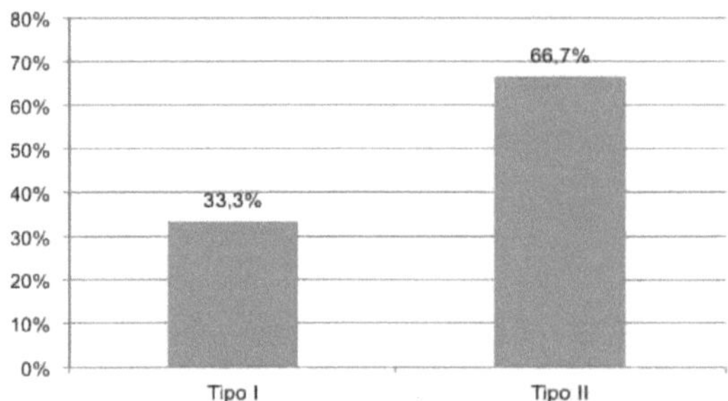

Figure 5.3 - Distribution of the sample according to Newton's classification

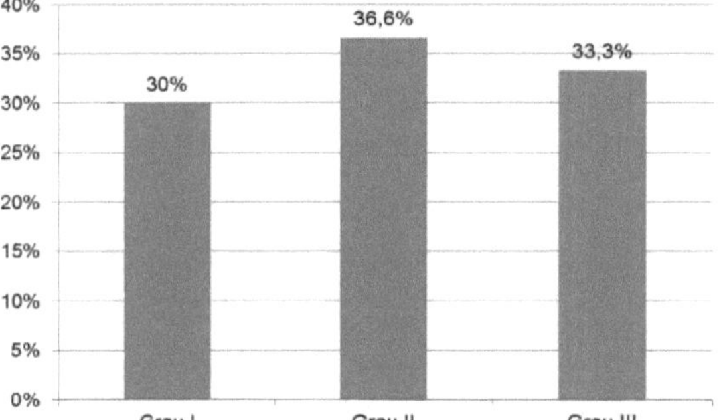

Figure 5.4 - Distribution of the sample according to the degree of erythema, before the intervention

5.3 CYTOLOGICAL FINDINGS OF THE PALATAL MUCOSA AND INTERNAL SURFACE OF MAXILLARY COMPLETE DENTURES BEFORE TREATMENT

Figure 5.5 shows the mean quantities of cytological cells in the palatal mucosa and on the inner surface of the prosthesis before treatment. It can be seen that the palatine mucosa showed greater quantities of superficial, intermediate, parabasal, basal, neutrophilic and mononuclear cells when compared to the cytological findings on the inner surface of the PT. However, the inner surface of the PT showed higher amounts of bacteria and fungi when compared to smears from the palatine mucosa. Of the 30 patients, 12 (40.0%) had hyphae on the palatine mucosa and on the inner surface of the PT, 11 (36.7%) had no hyphae on the mucosa, although they were present on the surface of the PT, while seven (23.3%) had no hyphae on the palatine mucosa and on the inner surface of the PT. This result suggested the active participation of the fungus in the aetiology of PE.

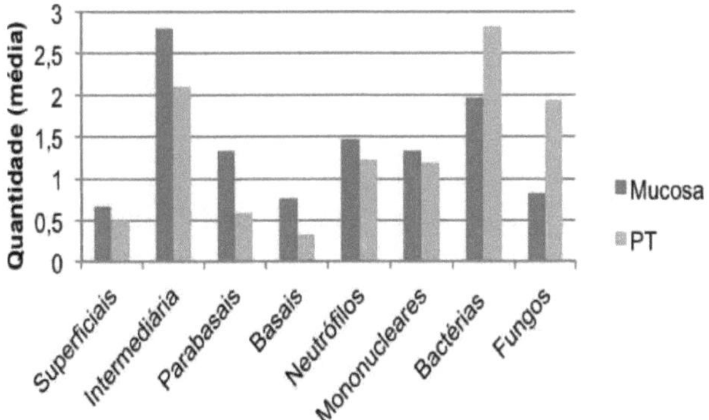

Figure 5.5 - Cytological findings of the palatine mucosa and the inner surface of the PT, before treatment

Figure 5.6 shows the cytological findings of the palatal mucosa of the inner surface of the PT before treatment.

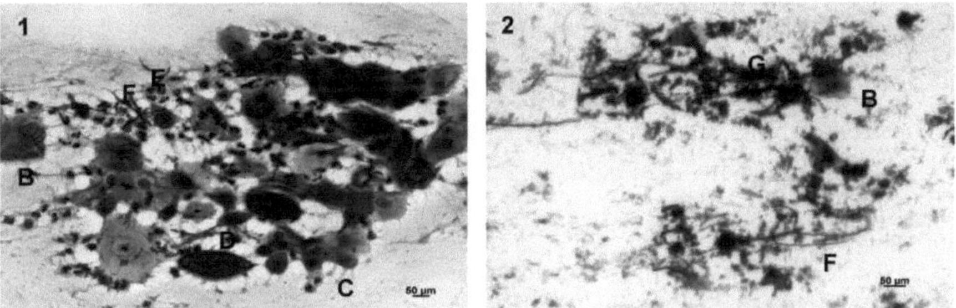

Figure 5.6 - (1) Cytological findings of the palatine mucosa before treatment, (2) Cytological findings of the inner surface of the PT before treatment: (A) superficial cells, (B) intermediate cells, (C) parabasal cells, (D) basal cells, (E) inflammatory cells, (F) hyphae, (G) biofilm

When applying the non-parametric Chi-squared test to compare the frequency of cytological findings on the palatal mucosa and the inner surface of the PT in the sample, we could see that there was a statistically significant difference for basal cells (p=0.343), as shown in table 5.3. However, there was a trend (p=0.063) towards an increase in the frequency of parabasal cells in the smears from the palatine mucosa and fungi in the smears from the inner surface of the PT.

Table 5.3 - Comparative values for the frequency of cytological findings on the palatine mucosa and the inner surface of the PT, before treatment

Variables	Palatine mucosa**	Jaw PT**	X2 calc	P
Surface	19	11	2,133	0,1441

Intermediate	30	30	0,000	1
Parabasais	26	14	3,600	0,0578
Basics	19	8	4,481	**0,0343***
Neutrophils	26	21	0,532	0,4658
Mononuclear	25	20	0,556	0,4561
Bacteria	28	30	0,069	0,7928
Fungi	12	23	3,457	0,063

*p<0,05
** number of patients
Critical X2 = 3.841

Table 5.4 shows the distribution, in mean (±SD), of the cytological findings of the smear from the palatine mucosa and the inner surface of the maxillary PT, respectively, according to Newton's classification before treatment. It can be seen from the smear of the palatine mucosa that Newton's type II had greater quantities of superficial, parabasal, basal, neutrophilic, mononuclear, bacterial and fungal cells. The same picture was repeated with regard to the number of cells on the internal surface of the maxillary PT, except for intermediate cells and bacteria, which had higher averages in Newton's type I.

Table 5.4 Cytological findings of the smear from the palatine mucosa and the inner surface of the maxillary PT, respectively, according to Newton's classification, before treatment

Variables	**Newton's classification**			
	Type 1		**Type II**	
	Mucosa	**EN**	**Mucosa**	**EN**
Surface	0,5+0,5	0,7±0,8	1,6±1,4	1,4+1,6
Intermediate	2,9+0,3	2±0,7	2,2±0,9	2,1+0,7
Parabasais	1,4+0,8	0,4±0,7	1,7±1,0	1,8+1,6
Basics	0,8±0,6	0,1±0,3	1,6±1,4	1,6+1,8
Neutrophils	1,1+0,7	0,8±0,8	2,1±1,0	2,0+1,3
Mononuclear	0,9+0,7	0,8±0,8	2,1±1,1	2,0+1,3
Bacteria	1,7+0,9	2,7±0,5	2,8±1,3	2,4+0,9
Fungi	0,8+1,2	1,4±1,3	1,6±1,6	2,3+1,2

5.4 INTERVENTION

5.4.1 Evaluation of the clinical effect of nystatin and propolis gel on the palatal mucosa

Table 5.5 shows the descriptive distribution of data on the degree of erythema of the palatal mucosa in patients before and after treatment with nystatin and propolis gel.

Table 5.5 - Distribution of patients according to the degree of erythema of the palatine mucosa before and after treatment with nystatin and propolis gel

Degree of erythema		**Nystatin**		**Propolis**	
		Day 0	**Day 14**	Day 0	**Day 14**
Grade 0	n	-	**7**	-	2
	%	-	46,7	-	13,3
Grade 1	n	4	5	5	**6**
	%	26,7	33,3	33,3	40,0
Grade II	n	6	2	5	2
	%	40,0	13,3	33,3	13,3
Grade III	n	5	1	5	5
	%	33,3	**6,7**	33,3	**33,3**
Total	n	15	15	15	15
	%	100	100	100	100

It can be seen that seven patients in the nystatin group showed a total reduction in erythema and five of those with moderate (grade II) and severe (grade III) inflammation showed a reduction in the degree of erythema on day 14. In the propolis gel group, two patients showed a total reduction in the degree of erythema on day 14, while those five patients who had severe inflammation (grade III) on day 0 showed no reduction in the degree of erythema at the end of treatment (day 14). For grade II there was a reduction in the degree of erythema compared to day 14.

Figure 5.7 shows the average degree of erythema of the palatal mucosa exposed to nystatin and propolis gel at the four analysis times. There was a gradual reduction in the average degree of erythema in the nystatin group when compared to the propolis gel group at the four analysis points. On day 5, the propolis gel group showed a reduction in the average from 2.0 to 1.1, however, on days 7 and 14 there was an increase in the average degree of erythema.

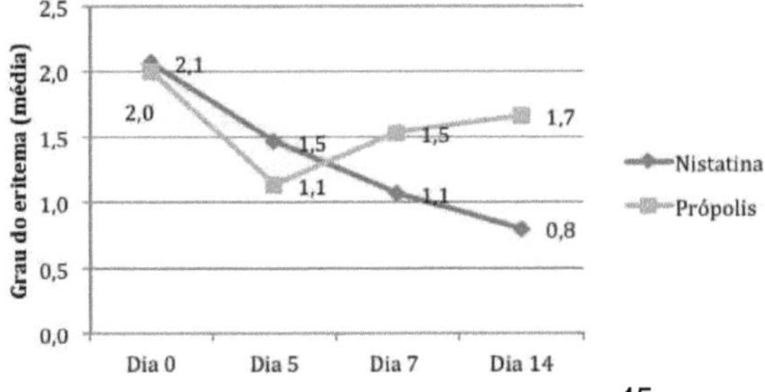

Figure 5.7 - Clinical efficacy of nystatin and propolis gel on the palatal mucosa

5.4.2 Cytological evaluation of the effect of nystatin and propolis gel on the palatal mucosa

Table 5.6 describes the cytological findings of the patients' palatal mucosa between the different times of the study analysis for both treatments. Friedman's non-parametric test was used to assess the cytological findings regarding the number of epithelial, inflammatory, bacterial and fungal cells at the four analysis times. A statistically significant difference (p=0.01) was found for the intermediate cells of the palatine mucosa of the patients who received nystatin. Once the difference had been found, multiple comparisons in rankings were carried out in order to show at which moments of the analysis the patient had received nystatin.

This difference was observed in the analysis. It was noted that there was a difference in the average ranking on day 0 and days 5 and 7, showing a decrease in the average ranking, i.e. an increase in the number of intermediate cells in the smear during these periods.

When we analysed the smear data from the patients who received the propolis gel, we noticed a statistically significant difference for surface cells (p=0.027), neutrophils (p=0.02) and bacteria (p=0.001) when compared at the four study moments. To check at which point there was a difference, we once again carried out multiple comparisons in ranking. The average ranking of superficial cells, neutrophils and bacteria increased at different points in the study, showing that there had been a decrease in the number of cells in the swab. For surface cells, the difference occurred between days 0 and 14 as well as 5 and 14; for neutrophils between days 0 and 7; 5 and 7 and 0 and 14. For bacteria, the difference was between day 0 and days 5, 7 and 14. These results suggest that propolis gel had some anti-inflammatory and antibacterial effect on the palatine mucosa.

Table 5.6 - Comparative values of the cytological findings of the patients' palate mucosa between the analysis times for both treatments

Treatment	Variables	0 days	5 days	7 days	14 days	F_{Fr}	p-value
Nystatin	Surface	2,40^{A}	2,53^{A}	2,40^{A}	2,67^{A}	0,84	0,481
Propolis		2,23^{A}	2,33^{A}	2.60^{A,B}	2,83^{B}	3,37	**0,027***
Nystatin	Intermediate	2,93^{B}	2,27^{A}	2,27^{A}	2.53^{A,B}	4,30	**0,010***
Propolis		2,20^{A}	2,33^{A}	2,70^{A}	2,77^{A}	2,66	0,060
Nystatin	Parabasais	2,70^{A}	2,30^{A}	2,43^{A}	2,57^{A}	0,70	0,557
Propolis		2,30^{A}	2,50^{A}	2,70^{A}	2,50^{A}	0,36	0,783
Nystatin	Basics	2,57^{A}	2,33^{A}	2,60^{A}	2,50^{A}	0,36	0,785
Propolis		2,40^{A}	2,43^{A}	2,73^{A}	2,43^{A}	0,55	0,650
Nystatin	Neutrophils	2,10^{A}	2,53^{A}	2,47^{A}	2,90^{A}	2,10	0,114
Propolis		2,07^{A}	2,27^{A,B}	2,93^{C}	2.73^{B,C}	3,67	**0,020***
Nystatin	Mononuclear	2,33^{A}	2,53^{A}	2,43^{A}	2,70^{A}	0,52	0,668
Propolis		2,10^{A}	2,30^{A}	2,80^{A}	2,80^{A}	2,36	0,085
Nystatin	Red blood cells	2,63^{A}	2,40^{A}	2,43^{A}	2,53^{A}	0,21	0,892
Propolis		2,50^{A}	2,23^{A}	2,47^{A}	2,80^{A}	0,89	0,452
Nystatin	Bacteria	2,67^{A}	2,40^{A}	2,37^{A}	2,57^{A}	0,24	0,870
Propolis		1,63^{A}	2,70^{B}	2,70^{B}	2,97^{B}	6,25	**0,001***
Nystatin	Fungi	2,33^{A}	2,23^{A}	2,63^{A}	2,80^{A}	2,24	0,098
Propolis		2,07^{A}	2,53^{A}	2,80^{A}	2,60^{A}	1,42	0,250

The higher the average ranking, the fewer the number of cells in the smear
Different letters (indices) indicate a statistical difference.
F_{Fr} (3.42) 5% (critical) = 2.83
Alpha = 0.05
*p<0,05

5.4.3 Cytological evaluation of the effect of nystatin and propolis gel on the internal surface of maxillary complete dentures

Table 5.7 shows the cytological findings of the inner surface of the PT between the study analysis times for both treatments. Friedman's non-parametric test showed that there was a statistically significant difference in the number of neutrophils (p=0.011), mononuclear cells (p=0.047) and fungi (p<0.001) in the patients who received nystatin between the four time points of the study. Multiple ranking comparisons were used to assess when the difference occurred. The average ranking of neutrophils, mononuclears and fungi showed a

increase in the averages between day 0 and days 5, 7 and 14, i.e. there was a decrease in these cells between the study periods.

When we evaluated the smears from the patients who received the propolis gel, we found that there was a significant difference in neutrophils (p=0.001) and mononuclear cells (p=0.001). The average ranking was used to assess the difference between the two time points. The average ranking showed that there was an increase in the average number of neutrophils and mononuclear cells between day 0 and days 7 and 14 and between day 5 and days 7 and 14, i.e. there was a reduction in the number of neutrophils and mononuclear cells in the PT smear. The same table also shows that there was a statistically significant difference for the bacteria of the patients who received the propolis gel (p<0.001), with the average ranking increasing between days 0 and days 5, 7 and 14 and between days 5 and 14, demonstrating that there was a decrease in the quantity of these cells.

There was a trend (p=0.06) towards a decrease in the number of parabasal cells and fungi in the palate mucosa smear of patients treated with propolis gel.

Table 5.7 - Comparative values of the cytological findings of the patients' palate mucosa between the analysis times for both treatments

Treatment	Variables	0 days	5 days	7 days	14 days	FR	p-value
Nystatin	Surface	2,50^{A}	2,47^{A}	2,47^{A}	2,57^{A}	0,10	0,96
Propolis		2,27^{A}	2,53^{A}	2,67^{A}	2,53^{A}	1,99	0,13
Nystatin	Intermediate	2,33^{A}	2,63^{A}	2,43^{A}	2,60^{A}	0,48	0,70
Propolis		2,30^{A}	2,30^{A}	2,70^{A}	2,70^{A}	1,91	0,14
Nystatin	Parabasais	2,17^{A}	2,63^{A}	2,67^{A}	2,53^{A}	1,73	0,18
Propolis		2,27^{A}	2,40^{A}	2,67^{A}	2,67^{A}	2,74	0,06
Nystatin	Basics	2,37^{A}	2,50^{A}	2,50^{A}	2,63^{A}	1,00	0,40
Propolis		2,37^{A}	2,63^{A}	2,50^{A}	2,50^{A}	0,79	0,51
Nystatin	Neutrophils	2,07^{A}	2,60^{B}	2,60^{B}	2,73^{B}	4,21	**0,011***
Propolis		1,97^{A}	2,23^{A}	2,90^{B}	2,90^{B}	6,49	**0,001***
Nystatin	Mononuclear	2,07^{A}	2,60^{B}	2,60^{B}	2,73^{B}	2,89	**0,047***
Propolis		1,97^{A}	2,23^{A}	2,90^{B}	2,90^{B}	6,49	**0,001***
Nystatin	Bacteria	2,37^{A}	2,47^{A}	2,60^{A}	2,57^{A}	0,18	0,91
Propolis		1,73^{A}	2,47^{B}	2.70^{B,C}	3,10^{C}	10,56	**2,66E-05***
Nystatin	Fungi	1,53^{A}	2,77^{B}	2,73^{B}	2,97^{B}	18,09	**1,09E-07***
Propolis		2,10^{A}	2,30^{A}	2,63^{A}	2,97^{A}	2,62	0,064

The higher the average ranking, the fewer the number of cells in the smear
Different letters (indices) indicate statistical difference.
F_{Fr}(3.42) 5% (critical) = 2.83
Alpha = 0.05
*p<0,05

5.4.4 Comparison of the cytological effect of nystatin and propolis gel on the palatal mucosa

Table 5.8 shows the comparative values of the effect of nystatin and propolis gel on the amount of bacteria and fungi in the swab of the palatal mucosa at the four time points of the study. The Mann-Whitney non-parametric test was used to compare the treatments.

Table 5.8 - Comparative values of the cytological effect of nystatin and propolis gel on the amount of bacteria and fungi in the palatal mucosa smear at the four study time points

Variables		Treatment	n	Average rank	p-value
Bacteria	5 days	Nystatin	15	14,33	0,445
		Propolis	15	16,67	
	7 days	Nystatin	15	13,60	0,213
		Propolis	15	17,40	
	14 days	Nystatin	15	13,70	0,238
		Propolis	15	17,30	
Fungi	5 days	Nystatin	15	16,83	0,347
		Propolis	15	14,17	
	7 days	Nystatin	15	17,83	**0,050***
		Propolis	15	13,17	
	14 days	Nystatin	15	18,50	**0,008***
		Propolis	15	12,50	

*p<0,05
The higher the average ranking, the fewer the number of cells in the smear

There was a statistically significant difference between nystatin and propolis gel for fungi on days 7 (p=0.050) and 14 (p=0.008), which suggests some antifungal effect of nystatin on the palatal mucosa.

Although no statistically significant difference was observed, it can be seen that the average ranking of propolis gel for bacteria showed an increase in values, from 16.67 to 17.30, i.e. the propolis gel reduced the amount of bacteria observed in the swab of the palate mucosa.

Figure 5.8 shows the cytological findings of the palatine mucosa before and after the intervention with nystatin and propolis gel.

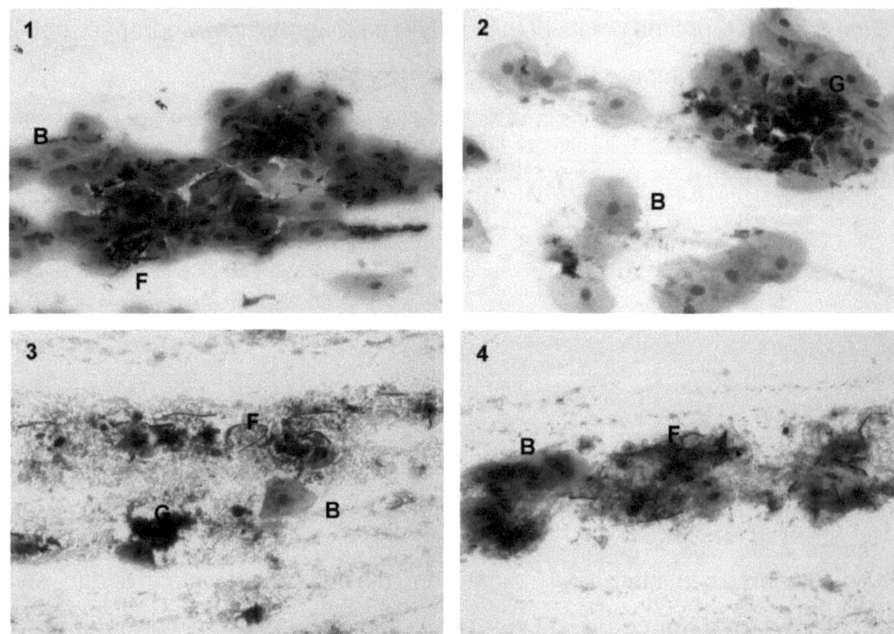

Figure 5.8 - (1) Cytological findings of the palatal mucosa before and after (2) treatment with nystatin; (3) Cytological findings of the palatal mucosa before and after (4) treatment with propolis gel: (A) superficial cells, (B) intermediate cells, (C) parabasal cells, (D) basal cells, (E) inflammatory cells, (F) hyphae, (G) bacteria;

5.4.5 Comparison of the cytological effect of nystatin and propolis gel on the internal surface of maxillary complete dentures

Table 5.9 shows comparative values for the effect of nystatin and propolis gel on the amount of bacteria and fungi present in the swab of the internal surface of the maxillary PT, obtained using the Mann-Whitney test. A statistically significant difference was found in the amount of fungi when comparing the effects of the treatments between days 5, 7 and 14, demonstrating the greater efficacy of nystatin in reducing the amount of fungi on the internal surface of the maxillary PT. There was no statistically significant difference in the number of bacteria when both interventions were compared. However, on day 14, there was a tendency for

decrease in the amount of bacteria in the swab of the internal surface of the maxillary PT treated with propolis gel when compared to nystatin (p=0.064).

Table 5.9 - Comparative values of the cytological effect of nystatin and propolis gel on the amount of bacteria and fungi on the internal surface of the maxillary PT at the four study moments

Variables	Treatments		n	Average rank	p-value
Bacteria	5 days	Nystatin	15	14,30	0,370
		Propolis	15	16,70	
	7 days	Nystatin	15	13,73	0,220
		Propolis	15	17,27	
	14 days	Nystatin	15	12,80	0,064
		Propolis	15	18,20	
Fungus	5 days	Nystatin	15	20,37	**0,001***
		Propolis	15	10,63	
	7 days	Nystatin	15	19,17	**0,011***
		Propolis	15	11,83	
	14 days	Nystatin	15	19,73	**0,003***
		Propolis	15	11,27	

*p<0,05
The higher the average ranking, the fewer the number of cells in the smear

Figure 5.9 shows the cytological findings of the inner surface of the PT before and after the intervention with nystatin and propolis gel.

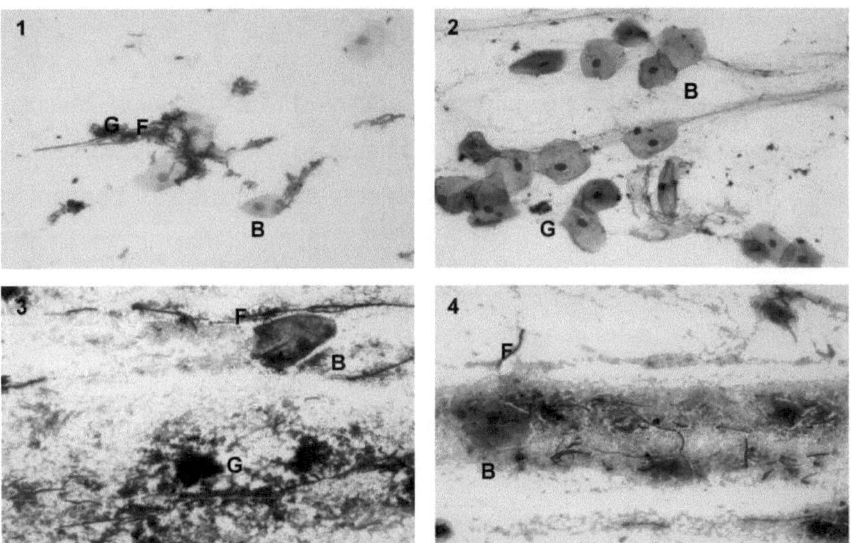

Figure 5.8 - (1) Cytological findings of the inner surface of the PT before and after (2) treatment with nystatin; (3) Cytological findings of the inner surface of the PT before and after (4) treatment with propolis gel: (A) superficial cells, (B) intermediate cells, (C) parabasal cells, (D) basal cells, (E) inflammatory cells, (F) hyphae, (G) bacteria

CHAPTER 6

DISCUSSION

Various proposals have emerged for the treatment of PE (63, 89, 90), but none have prevented the infection from recurring or the development of antifungal resistance (69, 100). Therefore, the development of new local therapies for the treatment of oral infectious diseases such as PE is of great relevance. Propolis has been studied for its pharmacological properties. Some studies have shown that propolis can have anti-inflammatory (22, 116), antibacterial (14, 118) and antifungal (16, 127, 129) activities, among others, which would justify its indication in the treatment of this infection. This was the aim of our study, which set out to evaluate the efficacy of propolis gel compared to nystatin suspension in the treatment of PE, by means of clinical and cytological analysis.

PE is a chronic inflammatory reaction of the palatine mucosa associated with the use of removable prostheses (8). In the study we set out to carry out, the prevalence of this inflammatory reaction was 23.1 per cent in elderly patients wearing TP. Arendorf and Walker (8) found that the prevalence of PE in PT wearers ranged from 11% to 67%. Freitas et al. (1) found that 57.2% of elderly PT users in a rural area in the west of Minas Gerais had PE. Pires et al. (38) found that the incidence of PE in PT users in Piracicaba was 50.6%. Marchini et al. (39) observed the occurrence of PE in 42.4% of PT users treated at the University of Mogi das Cruzes, SP.

Some authors have observed that this infection has a multifactorial aetiological character, and that poor hygiene and the continuous use of dentures have been identified as the most frequent causes associated with the appearance of the lesion (32, 45, 48, 69). Our study points to the use of dentures as the most prevalent risk factors for the onset of PE.

old ones associated with continuous use and the habit of sleeping with them.

Budtz-Jorgensen et al. (28) reported that old PTs are more difficult to clean due to their greater tendency to porosity, which favours colonisation by microorganisms. In addition, continuous use of dentures at night can reduce the protective effect of saliva, as well as the cleansing action of the tongue and oxygenation of the mucosa, which are important factors for the mucosa's resistance to mechanical and microbiological aggression exacerbated by their continuous use (34, 87). Abaci (49) adds that continuous use of PT increases the time the mucosa is exposed to the prosthesis biofilm.

PE is often asymptomatic and most patients report being unaware of the condition. In our study, 19 patients reported symptoms such as dry mouth (47.0%), unpleasant taste (30%), loss of taste (13%) and pain (10%). It is worth pointing out that not only PE may have contributed to the appearance of these symptoms, since advancing age may also be associated with systemic diseases, nutritional deficiencies, polypharmacy and changes in the quantity and quality of saliva. These factors, combined with the constant use of PT, could alter the oral microbiota.

Because it is a chronic inflammation, PE is characterised cytologically by the presence of superficial cells, intermediate cells, leucocytes and microorganisms (46, 58, 59, 135). This could be observed in our study, where the smear from the palatine mucosa showed mostly intermediate cells, as well as the presence of superficial, parabasal, basal cells, bacteria and fungi. These characteristics, according to Aguirre et al. (46), suggest that the inflammatory process accelerates the replacement of palatine mucosa epithelial cells in the presence of PE. We also observed the presence of neutrophils and mononuclear cells, as well as abundant bacteria in the mucosal smears. The presence of neutrophils, according to the same author, would be related to the positive culture of *Candida sp.,* while the large quantity of bacteria and the presence of yeast would contribute to the synergism observed between the biofilm *and Candida sp.*

Despite the low sensitivity and negative predictive value of exfoliative cytology for identifying fungal cells in smears, we found that 93.3% of patients had hyphae in the smear from the palatal mucosa or the inner surface of the PT, corroborating the results of Budtz-Jorgensen et al. (76), Aguirre (46) and Lemos (57) who found the hyphae form to be the most prevalent in the smears of patients with PE. We noticed that the smears from the inner surface of the PT, despite showing the same cytological findings as the mucosa, had a greater number of hyphae and bacteria when compared to the mucosa, although no significant difference was observed. These results lead us to believe that the colonisation of *Candida sp.* in the oral mucosa and on the surface of the PT can be considered the main etiological factor for the onset of PE, and that the PT can serve as a reservoir for the colonisation of bacteria and yeasts, as suggested by Pires et al. (38), Barbeau et al. (6), Emami et al. (66) and Campos et al. (83), since *Candida sp.* hyphae can adhere to the biofilm and/or penetrate the resin fissures (4).

We observed that type II PE, as well as being the most prevalent, also had a higher number of neutrophils, mononuclear cells, as well as bacteria and fungi in the mucosal smear when compared to type I. These findings corroborate those of Webb et al. (30), Barbeau et al. (6) and Lemos et al. (57) who stated that the extent of inflammation can determine the presence of fungal infection. Emami et al. (66) attributed this finding to the irritating action of the PT biofilm on the palatal mucosa, which can favour the installation of an inflammatory process as well as promoting the adhesion of pathogens.

Antifungal therapy is effective for treating inflammation associated with PE and is based on the pathogenic role of *Candida sp.* in this infection. The antifungals commonly used are imidazole compounds (miconazole gel) (110) and polyenes such as nystatin and amphotericin B (91). However, unless there is an improvement associated with the cleaning of the PTs and the reduction of *Candida sp.* on the surfaces of the prostheses, the effectiveness of antifungal treatment is limited, favouring the recurrence of PE within a short period of time.

There are few studies in the literature that have evaluated the effect of propolis in the treatment of PE. Therefore, the discussion in this paper is based on the few findings on the subject associated with the results found from *in vitro* studies.

In our study we used a 5% aqueous propolis extract gel, which consists of a mucoadhesive formulation that controls the release of the drug. We chose this formulation because of the difficulty encountered in the topical treatment of oral diseases where the constant salivary flow and mobility of the tissues involved mean that topical oral administration has the disadvantage of having an initial effect accompanied by a rapid decrease in concentration (9, 130).

Our results showed clinically that the nystatin suspension gradually reduced the degree of mucosal erythema at the four time points of the study, while the propolis gel showed a reduction in the average degree of erythema from 2.0 to 1.1 between days 0 and 5, and an increase in the degree of erythema between days 7 and 14. This implies that the propolis gel had a more powerful clinical effect, albeit quickly, when compared to nystatin, which showed an average reduction from 2.1 to 1.5 between days 0 and 5. This finding can be justified by the results found by Silva et al. (131) who demonstrated an increase in the surface roughness of the resin thanks to the deposition of the active ingredient of propolis on the resin. This was also observed in our study. We believe that the lack of dexterity of the elderly and the age of the PTs may have favoured the accumulation of propolis gel on the inner surface of the PTs, favouring reinfection of the mucosa with a consequent increase in the degree of erythema. In contrast, Santos et al. (25) showed that all patients treated with Miconazole (Daktarin® gel) and Brazilian propolis gel had clinical remission of palate oedema and erythema.

We also observed that propolis gel had some anti-inflammatory effect, since the number of neutrophils ($p=0.02$) in the mucosal smears, as well as neutrophils ($p=0.001$) and mononuclear cells ($p=0.001$) on the inner surface of the PT showed a statistically significant difference between days 0, 7 and 14, a fact that reinforces the findings in the literature (116).

The propolis gel showed some antibacterial effect, as the amount of bacteria in the mucosal swabs (p=0.001) and on the inner surface of the PT (p<0.001) showed a statistically significant reduction between the four study moments. Our findings are in line with reports in the literature (15, 118). On the other hand, Gomes et al. (130) observed that bacteria were more susceptible to 20% propolis ointment when compared to 1% tetracycline. It is believed that flavonoids act to inhibit bacterial RNA-polymerase or the bacterial cell membrane, causing functional and structural damage (118).

Many authors have studied the antifungal activity of propolis against *C. albicans*, and the ethanolic extract has been shown to be more effective (17, 108, 120). The ultrastructural findings seen in scanning electron micrographs suggest that the antifungal activity of propolis occurs due to changes in the fungal cell wall, which leads to an increase in volume and rupture of its cell membrane (108). We found no evidence of these findings in our study. However, Ota et al. (16) found a reduction in the number of *Candida sp.* in PT patients who used hydroalcoholic propolis extract. Dias et al. (128) demonstrated inhibition of the *in vitro* growth of *Candida sp.* exposed to ethanolic extracts of propolis. Molina et al. (129) showed that the glycolic extract of propolis had fungicidal capacity for all strains *of C. albicans.*

When comparing the treatments, we observed that nystatin showed a significant reduction in the amount of fungi (p>0.001), both in the swab of the palatal mucosa and on the inner surface of the PT. On the other hand, Santos et al. (24) observed a similar regression among PT patients with oral candidiasis who were treated with green propolis extract compared to the control group, which used nystatin.

Our results show that the aqueous extract of propolis used to make the gel had no antifungal effect. This was also confirmed by Dias et al. (128) who found that samples of aqueous propolis extracts showed little or no efficacy in inhibiting yeast growth *in vitro*. In addition, the aqueous propolis extract had a significantly smaller inhibition halo than nystatin in the microbiological tests. It is worth noting that the chemical composition of propolis varies according to the local flora, the region where it was collected, the period during which the resin was collected and the way the propolis was extracted, factors which can influence the concentration of flavonoids and, consequently, the pharmacological activities of propolis (114, 123); we believe that these may have been a factor in the negative antifungal effect of our gel.

Although several studies have shown antifungal and antibacterial activity for the ethanolic extract of propolis, we chose to use the aqueous extract of propolis since studies have reported that the ethanolic extract can cause irritation to the oral mucosa (9, 108). Another important factor found in our study, which may justify our results, was the 5% concentration of aqueous propolis extract used in the gel, given that Santos et al. (24, 25) used ethanolic propolis extract at 20 and 10%, respectively. However, Gomes et al. (130) showed that *Candida* strains were more susceptible to propolis at concentrations of 5, 10, 15 and 20 per cent than nystatin at 5 per cent. Furthermore, these same authors reported that the antimicrobial activity of propolis gel occurs in a dose-dependent manner. We used propolis gel for 14 days with four daily applications. Thus, we can suggest that our concentration of 5% and the dosage of propolis gel may also justify the negative antifungal effect in the treatment of PE.

The main limitation of this study was the lack of isolation of fungi using microbiological cultures. Despite this limitation, our results corroborate the relevant literature and the methodology applied demonstrates how important exfoliative cytology is for diagnosing PE, as well as aiding in the choice of treatment. However, more studies are needed to better evaluate the effect of propolis and its use in the treatment of PE.

CHAPTER 7

CONCLUSION

- The inner surface of the PT is a reservoir for the colonisation of micro-organisms, as it shows greater quantities of bacteria and fungi in the smear when compared to the palatine mucosa.
- Type II PE has a higher number of fungi and bacteria in the smear from the palatine mucosa and the inner surface of the PT.
- Nystatin showed a better clinical result compared to propolis gel, as there was a gradual reduction in the degree of erythema at all four points in the study.
- Propolis gel reduced the amount of bacteria present in the swab of the palatine mucosa and on the internal surface of the maxillary PT at the four time points of the study.
- Propolis gel reduced the number of neutrophils in the palatine mucosa at all four time points.
- Nystatin reduced the amount of fungi present in the swab from the inner surface of the maxillary PT at all four study moments.
- Nystatin significantly reduced the amount of fungi present in the swab of the palatine mucosa and the inner surface of the maxillary PT when compared to propolis gel.

REFERENCES[1]

1. Freitas JB, Gomez RS, De Abreu MH, Ferreira E Ferreira E. Relationship between the use of full dentures and mucosal alterations among elderly Brazilians. J Oral Rehabil. 2008 May;35(5):370-4.

2. Brazil. Ministry of Health. SB Brazil Project 2010. National Oral Health Survey: main results. Brasília-DF, 2011.

3. Cunha-Cruz J. One in 3 removable denture users in the United States

has denture stomatitis. J Evid Based Dent Pract. 2006 Jun;6(2): 197-8.

4. Ramage G, Tomsett K, Wickes BL, López-Ribot JL, Redding SW. Denture stomatitis: a role for Candida biofilms. Oral Surg Oral Med Oral Pathol Oral Radiol Endod. 2004 Jul;98(1):53-9.

5. Zissis A, Yannikakis S, Harrison A. Comparison of denture stomatitis prevalence in 2 population groups. Int J Prosthodont. 2006 Nov-Dec;19(6):621-5.

6. Barbeau J, Séguin J, Goulet JP, de Koninck L, Avon SL, Lalonde B, et al. Reassessing the presence of Candida albicans in denture-related stomatitis. Oral Surg Oral Med Oral Pathol Oral Radiol Endod. 2003 Jan;95(1):51-9.

7. Budtz-Jorgensen E, Mojon P, Rentsch A, Deslauriers N. Effects of an oral health programme on the occurrence of oral candidosis in a long-term care facility. Community Dent Oral Epidemiol. 2000 Apr;28(2): 141-9.

8. Arendorf TM, Walker DM. Denture stomatitis: a review. J Oral Rehabil. 1987 May;14(3):217-27.

9. Ceschel GC, Maffei P, Sforzini A, Lombardi Borgia S, Yasin A, Ronchi C. In vitro permeation through porcine buccal mucosa of caffeic acid phenetyl ester (CAPE) from a topical mucoadhesive gel containing propolis. Phytotherapy. 2002 Nov;73 Suppl 1:S44-52.

10. Lustosa S, Galindo A, Nunes L, Randau K, Rolim Neto P. Propolis: on chemistry and pharmacology. Braz Jl of Pharmacogn 2008;18(3):447-54.

11. Hayacibara MF, Koo H, Rosalen PL, Duarte S, Franco EM, Bowen WH, et al. In vitro and in vivo effects of isolated fractions of Brazilian propolis on caries development. J Ethnopharmacol. 2005 Oct; 101(1-3): 110-5.

12. Hu F, Hepburn HR, Li Y, Chen M, Radloff SE, Daya S. Effects of ethanol and water extracts of propolis (bee glue) on acute inflammatory animal models. J Ethnopharmacol. 2005 Sep;100(3):276-83.

13. Volpi N, Bergonzini G. Analysis of flavonoids from propolis by on-line HPLC-electrospray mass spectrometry. J Pharm Biomed Anal. 2006

Sep;42(3):354-61.

14. Menezes H, Bacci J, Oliveira S, Pagnocca F. Anti-bacterial properties of propolis and products containing propolis from Brazil. Apidologie. 1997;28:71 - 6.

15. Sforcin JM, Fernandes A, Jr, Lopes CA, Bankova V, Funari SR. Seasonal effect on Brazilian propolis antibacterial activity. J Ethnopharmacol. 2000 Nov;73(1-2):243-9.

16. Ota C, Unterkircher C, Fantinato V, Shimizu MT. Antifungal activity of propolis on different species of Candida. Mycoses. 2001 Nov;44(9-10):375-8.

17. Sawaya AC, Palma AM, Caetano FM, Marcucci MC, da Silva Cunha IB, Araújo CE, et al. Comparative study of in vitro methods used to analyse the activity of propolis extracts with different compositions against species of Candida. Lett Appl Microbiol. 2002;35(3):203-7.

18. Starzyk J, Scheller S, Szaflarski J, Moskwa M, Stojko A. Biological properties and clinical application of propolis. IL Studies on the antiprotozoan activity of ethanol extract of propolis. Arzneimittelforschung. 1977;27(6):1198-9.

19. Amoros M, Sauvager F, Girre L, Cormier M. In vitro anti-viral activity of propolis. Apidologie. 1992;23:231-40.

20. Grunberger D, Banerjee R, Eisinger K, Oltz E, Efros L, Caldwell M, et al. Preferential cytotoxicity on tumour cells by caffeic acid phenethyl esther isolated from propolis. Experientia. 1988;44:230-2.

21. Dimov V, Ivanovska N, Bankova V, Nikolov N, Popov S. Immunomodulatory action of propolis: IV. Prophylactic activity against Gram-negative infections and adjueffect of water soluble derivative. Vaccine. 1992;10:817-23.

22. Dobrowolski JW, Vohora SB, Sharma K, Shah SA, Naqvi SA, Dandiya PC. Antibacterial, antifungal, antiamoebic, anti-inflammatory and antipyretic studies on propolis bee products. J Ethnopharmacol. 1991 Oct;35(1):77-82.

23. Cheng P, Wong G. Honey bee propolis: prospects in medicine. Bee

World. 1996;77:8-15.

24. Santos VR, Pimenta FJ, Aguiar MC, do Carmo MA, Naves MD, Mesquita RA. Oral candidiasis treatment with Brazilian ethanol propolis extract. Phytother Res. 2005 Jul;19(7):652-4.

25. Santos VR, Gomes RT, de Mesquita RA, de Moura MD, França EC, de Aguiar EG, et al. Efficacy of Brazilian propolis gel for the management of denture stomatitis: a pilot study. Phytother Res. 2008 Nov;22(11): 1544-7

26. Crockett DN, O'Grady JF, Reade PC. Candida species and Candida albicans morphotypes in erythematous candidiasis. Oral Surg Oral Med Oral Pathol. 1992 May;73(5):559-63.

27. Cahn LR. Letter: Denture-related candidiasis. Oral Surg Oral Med Oral Pathol. 1976 Jan;41(1):59-60.

28. Budtz-Jorgensen E. Clinical aspects of Candida infection in denture wearers. J Am Dent Assoe. 1978 Mar;96(3):474-9.

29. Cross LJ, Bagg J, Wray D, Aitchison T. A comparison of fluconazole and itraconazole in the management of denture stomatitis: a pilot study. J Dent. 1998 Nov;26(8):657-64.

30. Webb BC, Thomas CJ, Willcox MD, Harty DW, Knox KW. Candida-associated denture stomatitis. Aetiology and management: a review. Part 1.

Factors influencing distribution of Candida species in the oral cavity. Aust Dent J. 1998 Feb;43(1):45-50.

31. Newton A. Denture sore mouth - a possible etiology. Br Dent J. 1962;112:357-60.

32. Budtz-Jorgensen E, Bertram U. Denture stomatitis. I. The etiology in relation to trauma and infection. Acta Odontol Scand. 1970 Mar;28(1):71-92.

33. Bergendal T, Isacsson G. A combined clinical, mycological and histological study of denture stomatitis. Acta Odontol Scand. 1983;41(1):33-44

34. Shulman JD, Rivera-Hidalgo F, Beach MM. Risk factors associated with denture stomatitis in the United States. J Oral Pathol Med. 2005 Jul;34(6):340-6.

35. Kovac-Kavcic M, Skaleric U. The prevalence of oral mucosal lesions in a population in Ljubljana, Slovenia J Oral Pathol Med. 2000;28:331-5.

36. Mumcu G, Cimilli H, Sur H, Hayran O, Atalay T. Prevalence and distribution of oral lesions: a cross-sectional study in Turkey. Oral Dis. 2005 Mar;11(2):81-7. PubMed PMID: 15752080. eng.

37. Garcia-Pola Vallejo MJ, Martinez Diaz-Canel Al, Garcia Martin JM, Gonzalez Garcia M. Risk factors for oral soft tissue lesions in an adult Spanish population. Community Dent Oral Epidemiol. 2002 Aug;30(4):277-85.

38. Pires FR, Santos EB, Bonan PR, De Almeida OP, Lopes MA. Denture stomatitis and salivary Candida in Brazilian edentulous patients. J Oral Rehabil. 2002 Nov;29(11):1115-9.

39. Marchini L, Tamashiro E, Nascimento DF, Cunha VP. Self-reported denture hygiene of a sample of edentulous attendees at a University dental clinic and the relationship to the condition of the oral tissues. Gerodontology. 2004 Dec;21(4):226-8.

40. da Silva HF, Martins-Filho PR, Piva MR. Denture-related oral mucosal lesions among farmers in a semi-arid Northeastern Region of Brazil. Med Oral Pathol Oral Cir Bucal. 2011 Sep 1;16(6):e740-4.

41. Ferreira RC, Magalhães CS, Moreira AN. Oral mucosal alterations among the institutionalised elderly in Brazil. Braz Oral Res. 2010 Jul-Sep;24(3):296-302.

42. Budtz-Jorgensen E, Lõe H. Chlorhexidine as a denture disinfectant in the treatment of denture stomatitis. Scand J Dent Res. 1972;80(6):457-64.

43. Figueiral MH, Azul A, Pinto E, Fonseca PA, Branco FM, Scully C. Denture-related stomatitis: Identification of aetiological and predisposing factors - a large cohort. J Oral Rehabil. 2007 Jun;34(6):448-55.

44. Pinto E, Ribeiro IC, Ferreira NJ, Fortes CE, Fonseca PA, Figueiral MH. Correlation between enzyme production, germ tube formation and susceptibility to fluconazole in Candida species isolated from patients with denture-related stomatitis and control individuals. J Oral Pathol Med. 2008 Nov;37(10):587-92.

45. Zissis A, Yannikakis S, Harrison A. Comparison of denture stomatitis prevalence in 2 population groups. Int J Prosthodont. 2006 Nov-Dec;19(6):621-5.

46. Aguirre JM, Verdugo F, Zamacona JM, Quindos G, Ponton J. Cytological changes in oral mucosa in denture stomatitis. Gerodontology. 1996 Jul;13(1):63-7.

47. MacEntee MI, Glick N, Stolar E. Age, gender, dentures and oral mucosal disorders. Oral Dis. 1998 Mar;4(1):32-6.

48. Kossioni AE. The prevalence of denture stomatitis and its predisposing conditions in an older Greek population. Gerodontology. 2011 Jun;28(2):85-90.

49. Abaci O, Haliki-Uztan A, Ozturk B, Toksavul S, Ulusoy M, Boyacioglu H. Determining Candida spp. incidence in denture wearers. Mycopathologia. 2010 May;169(5):365-72.

50. Espinoza I, Rojas R, Aranda W, Gamonal J. Prevalence of oral mucosal lesions in elderly people in Santiago, Chile. J Oral Pathol Med. 2003 Nov;32(10):571-5.

51. Al-Dwairi ZN. Prevalence and risk factors associated with denture-related stomatitis in healthy subjects attending a dental teaching hospital in North Jordan. J Ir Dent Assoe. 2008 2008 Apr-May;54(2):80-3.

52. Baran I, Nalçaci R. Self-reported denture hygiene habits and oral tissue conditions of complete denture wearers. Arch Gerontol Geriatr. 2009 2009 Sep-Oct;49(2):237-41.

53. Evren BA, Uludamar A, I§eri U, Ozkan YK. The association between socioeconomic status, oral hygiene practice, denture stomatitis and oral status in elderly people living different residential homes. Arch Gerontol Geriatr. 2011 Nov-Dec;53(3):252-7.

54. Mandali G, Sener ID, Turker SB, Ulgen H. Factors affecting the distribution and prevalence of oral mucosal lesions in complete denture wearers. Gerodontology. 2011 Jun;28(2):97-103.

55. Scalercio M, Valente T, Israel MS, Ramos ME. Prophetic stomatitis versus candidiasis: diagnosis and treatment. RGO. 2007;55(4):395-8.

56. Budtz-Jorgensen E. Etiology, pathogenesis, therapy, and prophylaxis of oral yeast infections. Acta Odontol Scand. 1990 Feb;48(1):61-9.

57. Lemos MMC, Miranda JLD, Souza MSGDS. Clinic, microbiologic and histophatologic study of the denture stomatitis. Rev Bras Patol Oral. 2003;2(1):3-10.

58. Kaaber S, Bertram U. Cytology of the inflammatory exudate in denture stomatitis. Scand J Dent Res. 1971;79(2):81-91.

59. Ritchie GM, Fletcher AM, Main DM, Prophet AS. The etiology, exfoliative cytology, and treatment of denture stomatitis. J Prosthet Dent. 1969 Aug;22(2): 185-200.

60. Aguirre Urizar JM, Zamacona Gros JM, Kutz Aramburu R, Echebarria Goicouria MA. Denture stomatitis. 2. Histopathological, diagnostic and therapeutic aspects. Rev Actual Odontoestomatol Esp. 1990 Jun;50(394):31-7.

61. Williams DW, Lewis MA. Isolation and Identification of Candida from the oral cavity. Oral Dis. 2000 Jan;6(1):3-11.

62. Biocina-Lukenda D, Gregurek-Novak T, Cekic-Arambasin A. Denture stomatitis associated with allergic reaction to teeth prostheses. J Eur Acad Dermatol Venereol. 2004 Mar;18(2):227-9.

63. Bergendal T. Status and treatment of denture stomatitis patients: a 1-year follow-up study. Scand J Dent Res. 1982 Jun;90(3):227-38.

64. Budtz-Jorgensen E, Milton Knudsen A. Chlorhexidine gel and Steradent employed in cleaning dentures. Acta Odontol Scand. 1978;36(2):83-7.

65. Gonsalves WC, Wrightson AS, Henry RG. Common oral conditions in older persons. Am Fam Physician. 2008 Oct;78(7):845-52.

66. Emami E, Séguin J, Rompré PH, de Koninck L, de Grandmont P, Barbeau J. The relationship of myceliated colonies of Candida albicans with denture stomatitis: an in vivo/in vitro study. Int J Prosthodont. 2007 Sep-Oct;20(5):514-20.

67. Webb BC, Thomas CJ, Willcox MD, Harty DW, Knox KW. Candida-associated denture stomatitis. Aetiology and management: a review. Part 2. Oral diseases caused by Candida species. Aust Dent J. 1998 Jun;43(3):160-6.

68. Arendorf TM, Walker DM. Oral candidal populations in health and disease. Br Dent J. 1979 Nov;147(10):267-72.

69. Gendreau L, Loewy ZG. Epidemiology and etiology of denture stomatitis. J Prosthodont. 2011 Jun;20(4):251-60.

70. Coco BJ, Bagg J, Cross LJ, Jose A, Cross J, Ramage G. Mixed Candida albicans and Candida glabrata populations associated with the pathogenesis of denture stomatitis. Oral Microbiol Immunol. 2008 Oct;23(5):377-83.

71. Kulak-Ozkan Y, Kazazoglu E, Arikan A. Oral hygiene habits, denture cleanliness, presence of yeasts and stomatitis in elderly people. J Oral Rehabil. 2002 Mar;29(3):300-4.

72. Kulak Y, Arikan A, Kazazoglu E. Existence of Candida albicans and microorganisms in denture stomatitis patients. J Oral Rehabil. 1997 Oct;24(10):788-90.

73. de Oliveira CE, Gasparoto TH, Dionísio TJ, Porto VC, Vieira NA, Santos CF, et al. Candida albicans and denture stomatitis: evaluation of its presence in the lesion, prosthesis, and blood. Int J Prosthodont. 2010 Mar-Apr;23(2): 158-9.

74. Carvalho de Oliveira TR; Frigerio MLMA; Yamada MCM; Birman EG. Evaluation of prophetic stomatitis in denture wearers. Pesqui Odontol Bras 2000 jul/set;14(3):219-224.

75. Cahn L. The denture sore mouth. Ann Dent 1936;3:33-6.

76. Budtz-Jorgensen E. The role of Candida albicans in the development of stomatitis in denture wearers. Med Hyg (Geneve). 1975 Oct;33(1164):1434-5.

77. Zomorodian K, Haghighi NN, Rajaee N, Pakshir K, Tarazooie B, Vojdani M, et al. Assessment of Candida species colonisation and denture-related stomatitis in complete denture wearers. Med Mycol. 2011 Feb;49(2):208-11.

78. Pereira-Cenci T, Del Bei Cury AA, Crielaard W, Ten Cate JM. Development of Candida-associated denture stomatitis: new insights. J Appl Oral Sei. 2008 Mar-Apr;16(2):86-94.

79. Radford DR, Challacombe SJ, Walter JD. Denture plaque and adherence of Candida albicans to denture-base materials in vivo and in vitro. Crit Rev Oral Biol Med. 1999;10(1):99-116.

80. Serrano-Granger C, Cerero-Lapiedra R, Campo-Trapero J, Del Río-Highsmith J. In Vitro Study of the Adherence of Candida Albicans to Acrylic Resins: Relationship to Surface Energy. Int J Prosthodont 2005;18:392-8.

81. Yoshijima Y, Murakami K, Kayama S, Liu D, Hirota K, Ichikawa T, et al. Effect of substrate surface hydrophobicity on the adherence of yeast and hyphal Candida. Mycoses. 2010 May;53(3):221-6.

82. Elguezabal N, Maza JL, Dorronsoro S, Pontón J. Whole Saliva has a Dual Role on the Adherence of Candida albicans to Polymethylmethacrylate. Open Dent J. 2008;2:1-4.

83. Campos MS, Marchini L, Bernardes LA, Paulino LC, Nobrega FG. Biofilm microbial communities of denture stomatitis. Oral Microbiol Immunol. 2008 Oct;23(5):419-24.

84. Coco BJ, Bagg J, Cross LJ, Jose A, Cross J, Ramage G. Mixed Candida albicans and Candida glabrata populations associated with the pathogenesis of denture stomatitis. Oral Microbiol Immunol. 2008 Oct;23(5):377-83.

85. Vanden Abbeele A, de Meei H, Ahariz M, Perraudin JP, Beyer I,

Courtois P. Denture contamination by yeasts in the elderly. Gerodontology. 2008 Dec;25(4):222-8.

86. Farah CS, Lynch N, McCullough MJ. Oral fungal infections: an update for the general practitioner. Aust Dent J. 2010 Jun;55 Suppl 1:48-54

87. Emami E, de Grandmont P, Rompré PH, Barbeau J, Pan S, Feine JS. Favouring trauma as an etiological factor in denture stomatitis. J Dent Res. 2008 May;87(5):440-4

88. Dagistan S, Aktas AE, Caglayan F, Ayyildiz A, Bilge M. Differential diagnosis of denture-induced stomatitis, Candida, and their variations in patients using complete denture: a clinicai and mycological study. Mycoses. 2009 May;52(3):266-71

89. Webb BC, Thomas CJ, Harty DW, Willcox MD. Effectiveness of two methods of denture sterilisation. J Oral Rehabil. 1998 Jun;25(6):416-23.

90. Walker DM, Stafford GD, Huggett R, Newcombe RG. The treatment of denture-induced stomatitis. Evaluation of two agents. Br Dent J. 1981 Dec;151(12):416-9.

91. Salerno C, Pascale M, Contaldo M, Esposito V, Busciolano M, Milillo L, Guida A, Petruzzi M, Serpico R. Candida-associated denture stomatitis. Med Oral Pathol Oral Cir Bucal. 2011 Mar;16(2):e139-43.

92. Budtz-Jorgensen E, Bertram U. Denture stomatitis. II. The effect of antifungal and prosthetic treatment. Acta Odontol Scand. 1970 Jun;28(3):283-304.

93. Bergendal T, Isacsson G. Effect of nystatin in the treatment of denture stomatitis. Scand J Dent Res. 1980 Oct;88(5):446-54.

94. Dorocka-Bobkowska B, Konopka K, Dúzgúneç N. Influence of antifungal polyenes on the adhesion of Candida albicans and Candida glabrata to human epithelial cells in vitro. Arch Oral Biol. 2003 Dec;48(12):805-14.

95. Geerts GA, Stuhlinger ME, Basson NJ. Effect of an antifungal denture liner on the saliva yeast count in patients with denture stomatitis: a pilot

study. J Oral Rehabil. 2008 Sep;35(9):664-9.

96. Parvinen T, Kokko J, Yli-Urpo A. Micotiazole lacquer cotnpared with gel in treattnetit of denture stotnatitis. Scand J Dent Res 1994;102:361-6.

97. Dias AP, Samaranayake LP, Lee MT. Miconazole lacquer in the treatment of denture stomatitis: clinical and microbiological findings in Chinese patients. Clin Oral Investig. 1997 Feb;1(1):47-52.

98. Chow CK, Matear DW, Lawrence HP. Efficacy of antifungal agents in tissue conditioners in treating candidiasis. Gerodontology. 1999 Dec; 16(2): 110-8.

99. Budtz-Jorgensen E, Holmstrup P, Krogh P. Fluconazole in the treatment of Candida-associated denture stomatitis. Antimicrob Agents Chemother. 1988 Dec;32(12): 1859-63.

100. Kulak Y, Arikan A, Delibalta N. Comparison of three different treatment methods for generalised denture stomatitis. J Prosthet Dent. 1994 Sep;72(3):283-8.

101. Arikan A, Kulak Y, Kadir T. Comparison of different treatment methods for localised and generalized simple denture stomatitis. J Oral Rehabil. 1995 May;22(5):365-9.

102. Cross LJ, Bagg J, Aitchison TC. Efficacy of the cyclodextrin liquid preparation of itraconazole in treatment of denture stomatitis: comparison with itraconazole capsules. Antimicrob Agents Chemother. 2000 Feb;44(2):425-7

103. Cross LJ, Williams DW, Sweeney CP, Jackson MS, Lewis MA, Bagg J. Evaluation of the recurrence of denture stomatitis and Candida colonisation in a small group of patients who received itraconazole. Oral Surg Oral Med Oral Pathol Oral Radiol Endod. 2004 Mar;97(3):351-8.

104. Koray M, Ak G, Kurklu E, Issever H, Tanyeri H, Kulekci G, et al. Fluconazole and/or hexetidine for management of oral candidiasis associated with denture-induced stomatitis. Oral Dis. 2005 Sep;11(5):309-13.

105. Dorocka-Bobkowska B, Konopka K. Susceptibility of candida isolates

from denture-related stomatitis to antifungal agents in vitro. Int J Prosthodont. 2007 Sep-Oct;20(5):504-6.

106. Calixto JB. Efficacy, safety, quality control, marketing and regulatory guidelines for herbal medicines (phytotherapeutic agents). Braz J Med Biol Res. 2000 Feb;33(2): 179-89.

107. Agra M, Freitas P, Barbosa-Filho J. Synopsis of the plants known as medicinal and poisonous in Northeast of Brazil. Rev Bras Farmacogn. 2007;17(1):114-40.

108. Casaroto AR, Lara VS. Phytomedicines for Candida-associated denture stomatitis. Fitoterapia. 2010 Jul;81(5):323-8.

109. Vasconcelos LC, Sampaio MC, Sampaio FC, Higino JS. Use of Púnica granatum as an antifungal agent against candidosis associated with denture stomatitis. Mycoses. 2003 Jun;46(5-6): 192-6.

110. Amanlou M, Beitollahi JM, Abdollahzadeh S, Tohidast-Ekrad Z. Miconazole gel compared with Zataria multiflora Boiss. gel in the treatment of denture stomatitis. Phytother Res. 2006 Nov;20(11):966-9.

111. Catalan A, Pacheco JG, Martinez A, Mondaca MA. In vitro and in vivo activity of Melaleuca alternifolia mixed with tissue conditioner on Candida albicans. Oral Surg Oral Med Oral Pathol Oral Radiol Endod. 2008 Mar;105(3):327-32.

112. Paiva, ALCD, Ribeiro, AR, Pereira, VJ, Oliveira NMC. Clinical and laboratory evaluation of Uncaria tomentosa (Cat's Claw) gel on oral candidosis. Rev Bras de Farmacogn. 2009;19(2A):423-8.

113. Pereira A, Seixas F, Aquino Neto F. Propolis: 100 years of research and its future prospects. Quim Nova 2002;25:321-6.

114. Park YK, Alencar SM, Aguiar CL. Botanical origin and Chemical composition of Brazilian propolis. J Agric Food Chem. 2002 Apr 24;50(9):2502-6.

115. Marcucci M. Biological and therapeutic properties of the chemical constituents of propolis.Quim Nova 1996;19:529-36.

116. Burdock GA. Review of the biological properties and toxicity of bee propolis (propolis). Food Chem Toxicol. 1998 Apr;36(4):347-63.

117. Bankova V. Chemical diversity of propolis and the problem of standardisation. J Ethnopharmacol. 2005 Aug 22; 100(1-2): 114-7.

118. Uzel A, Sorkun K, Oncag O, Cogulu D, Gencay O, Salih B. Chemical compositions and antimicrobial activities of four different Anatolian propolis samples. Microbiol Res. 2005; 160(2): 189-95.

119. Mantovani R, Rall V, Batalha J, Fernandes A, Fernandes Júnior A. Anti-coagulase-negative Staphylococcus activity of ethanolic extracts of propolis from two Brasilian regions and synergism with antimicrobial drugs by E-Test method. J of venomous animals and toxins incluing tropical diseases. 2008;14:357-65.

120. Castaldo S, Capasso F. Propolis, an old remedy used in modern medicine. Fitoterapia. 2002 Nov;73 Suppl 1:S1-6.

121. Popova M, Silici S, Kaftanoglu O, Bankova V. Antibacterial activity of Turkish propolis and its qualitative and quantitative Chemical composition. Phytomedicine. 2005 Mar;12(3):221-8.

122. Ghisalberti E. Propolis: a review. Bee World. 1979;60:59-84.

123. Park YK, Koo MH, Abreu JA, Ikegaki M, Cury JA, Rosalen PL. Antimicrobial activity of propolis on oral microorganisms. Curr Microbiol. 1998 Jan;36(1):24-8.

124. Antunes R, Catao R, Cevallos B. Antimicrobial activity of propolis. Rev Bras de Farm. 1996;77:15-8.

125. Longhini R, Raksa S, Oliveira A, Svidzinski T, Franco S. Obtaining propolis extracts under different conditions and evaluating their antifungal activity. Rev Bras Farmacogn. 2007:388-95.

126. Ota C, Unterkircher C, Fantinato V, Shimizu MT. Antifungal activity of propolis on different species of Candida. Mycoses. 2001 Nov;44(9-10):375-8.

127. D'Auria FD, Tecca M, Scazzocchio F, Renzini V, Strippoli V. Effect of

propolis on virulence factors of Candida albicans. J Chemother. 2003 Oct;15(5):454-60.

128. Dias S, Gomes R, Santiago W, Paula A, Cortês M, Santos V. Antifungal activity of commercial ethanolic and aqueous extracts of Brazilian propolis against Candida spp. Rev Ciênc Farm Básica Apl. 2007;28(3):259-63.

129. Molina FP MM, Perrela FA, Oliveira LD, Junqueira JC, Jorge AOC. Propolis, salvia, calendula and castor - antifungal activity of natural extracts on Candida albicans strains. Cienc Odontol Bras 2008 11(2):86-93.

130. Gomes R, Teixeira K, Cortês M, Santos V. Antimicrobial activity of a propolis adhesive formulation on different oral pathogens. Braz J Oral Sei. 2007:6(22): 1387-91.

131. da Silva WJ, Rached RN, Rosalen PL, Del bei Cury AA. Effects of nystatin, fluconazole and propolis on poly(methyl methacrylate) resin surface. Braz Dent J. 2008; 19(3): 190-6.

132. Brazil. Resolution 196, of 10 October 1996. Approves guidelines and regulatory norms for research involving human beings. In: Saúde BICNd, editor. 1996.

133. Hulley S, Cummings S, Browner W, Grady D, Newman T. Designing Clinical Research: An Epidemiological Approach. 3 ed. Porto Alegre; Editora Artmed, 2008.

134. Folstein M. Mini-mental and son. Int J Geriatr Psychiatry. 1998; 12:290-4.

135. Olsen I, Stenderup A. Clinical-mycologic diagnosis of oral yeast infections. Acta Odontol Scand. 1990 Feb;48(1):11-8.

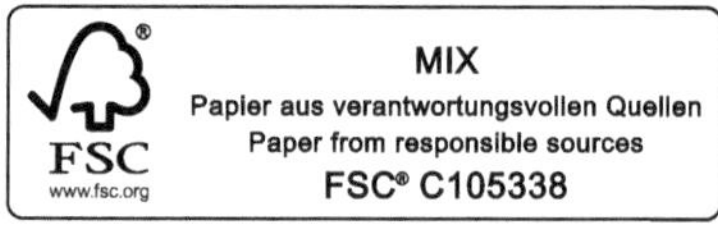

Printed by Books on Demand GmbH, Norderstedt / Germany